The Unassisted Baby

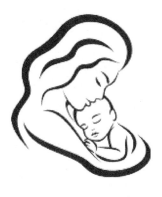

A Do-It-Yourself Guide to Pregnancy and Childbirth

3rd Edition, March 2021.

ISBN-13: 978-1-7350935-6-7

This book is dedicated to my children.

Without you, I would have never written about childbirth.

Contents

Preface

I am the mother of five beautiful children. Like many other women, I started motherhood in the more "traditional" way. My first child was born in a hospital with an OB/GYN "performing the delivery". I even had an epidural.

Needless to say, I didn't enjoy the experience. I couldn't feel the actual birth, and I had to be without my daughter right afterwards, because she had to be evaluated. It took me several weeks to bond with her, and I was disappointed with my unnatural birth experience.

My second daughter was born in the bathtub at a birth center with a midwife. There was a world of difference between this birth and the first. I fell in love with her immediately. Best of all, the midwives actively involved me in every decision regarding her care during and after birth.

My third child was our first boy and my first unassisted birth. The pregnancy and birth journey with him inspired me to write this book.

With my fourth baby, I had an unassisted pregnancy and an unassisted birth. At almost 44 weeks gestation, I finally gave birth to my second son in the hands-and-knees position.

My fifth child, the tie-breaker girl, was also born unassisted at home, despite meconium in the water. I'll share my full birth stories at the back of this book with you.

Every birth is different. Even my three unassisted births were not alike. But my good birth experiences have several things in common: a safe birthing space, people I trust, and the belief in my ability to give birth naturally.

My wish for you is to have the childbirth experience you want. If an unassisted birth is right for you, then I want to help you have one.

Introduction

"Your body is not a lemon!"

- Ina May Gaskin

Congratulations! If you're reading this book, chances are you're pregnant or planning on becoming pregnant. You may even read this book because someone told you about it, and it spiked your curiosity.

There are a lot of different books on childbirth available. Most of them, including the well-known bestseller "What to Expect When You're Expecting" by Heidi Murkoff and Sharon Mazel, focus on traditional prenatal care and childbirth in our Western world.

Unfortunately, traditional prenatal care and childbirth are fear-based. The pregnant woman is encouraged to seek medical care, often even before conception. We expect pregnant women to find a caregiver and consult him or her throughout the process. As promising as it sounds, choosing a caregiver is usually where the autonomy of the pregnant woman ends.

Once a caregiver is chosen, many women create birth plans. Often, they're told to be flexible, because their medical caregivers won't (or don't want to) meet their expectations. Unfortunately, most women are not truly in charge of their pregnancy and childbirth experience, but willingly submit to the authority of medically trained personnel. Therefore, the books merely explain what could happen and why, preparing women for potential complications.

Most traditional pregnancy and childbirth literature doesn't emphasize women's ability to birth their own babies. Fortunately, there are a few exceptions. For example, Ina May Gaskin's book illustrates how a woman's body can naturally give birth as long as nobody interferes with the process.

My book is also a little different. Based on my personal experience with three different types of births, I am heavily biased towards a natural approach to childbirth. I believe this is the way we should have our babies.

In a lot of cultures around the world, having a baby is still a natural occurrence versus a heavily medically supervised one. Pregnancy and childbirth aren't considered alarming or worrisome. Instead, both are normal processes. In those cultures, which are often far removed from Western medicine, nobody questions the woman's ability to safely grow her baby in her uterus and to give birth to him when it's time.

Unfortunately, modern medicine does not have the same faith in women's bodies. As highly developed as humans are, we are the only species who cannot or will not give birth without professional assistance. Most of us are so far removed from nature we don't trust our own bodies to accomplish what they were designed to do.

Have you ever witnessed one of your pets or farm animals give birth? You may have noticed that the mother retreats and gives birth on her own, without alerting the family, the media, or a doctor.

We can do this, too.

I went from being an uninformed, first-time mom who did all the regular things (induced labor with epidural at a hospital) to having a baby without help (my third, fourth, and fifth babies). You can find my personal birth stories at the end of this book. I hope they inspire you and show you that you can do this, too.

While unassisted childbirth is on the rise, most women don't even know they have this option. Many freebirthers don't choose an unassisted birth until their second or subsequent pregnancy. And while your body can birth alone, an unassisted childbirth requires more preparation than any other type of birth.

Why I Wrote This Book

I'm a firm proponent of making educated decisions regarding your own health, not just during pregnancy. Being pregnant and having a baby is not like having a disease. You're not sick. If you normally don't go to the doctor when you're healthy, why would you go to the doctor just because you're pregnant? After all, pregnancy and childbirth are both natural processes.

Most likely, you conceived this baby alone with your partner. Similarly, your body knows how to take care of your baby and grow it safely inside your uterus. This is true even if you don't understand the entire process. You may not know exactly how your digestive system works, but yet it continues to function just fine.

In addition to growing a baby in your uterus, your body knows how to birth your baby. As a first-time mother, you may not know what to expect, and it's perfectly fine to have supportive birth attendants. Your doctor's or midwife's goal should be to help you do it on your own. But contrary to popular belief, having a natural birth *does not require* a birth attendant with a medical degree. In fact, having a medically trained birth attendant can even prevent you from having a natural birth.

How to Use This Book

This book covers basic information about natural childbirth, including prenatal care, pregnancy symptoms, labor, complications at birth, postpartum care for you, caring for your newborn, and a guide for fathers. I organized the topics based on the sequence of events (for example, pregnancy comes before labor and childbirth). And while I intend this book to be read from front to back, you can certainly skip around to the chapters you need.

While I tried to paint an accurate picture of pregnancy and childbirth and answer any questions you may have, this may not be a complete resource. I absolutely encourage you to do more research on your own and talk to medical professionals, if you want to. Just be aware that not every medical professional will be supportive of your decision to give birth unassisted, nor will some of your family members. Fortunately, childbirth is not inherently dangerous, even though many people seem to think so.

I want you to live with an empowered mindset. Throughout the book, I am trying to help you build just such a mindset. I explain the process of childbirth in detail, giving you most of the knowledge you need to safely give birth to your own baby. I will show you how you're capable of having a baby, even if you still need to find more answers after reading this book.

I realize you may have already read many other books on childbirth. However, I want this book to be easy to understand for everybody, including your partner. Therefore, when I use medical terms related to childbirth, I often explain them within the text. Please skip any explanations you don't need.

Warning!

I'm not a medical professional, nor do I claim to be one. I've researched the information in these pages as carefully as possible. I base some of it on my personal experience and the experience of others.

Most healthy women today can have a natural childbirth, but nobody (doctor, midwife, or layperson) can guarantee a positive outcome. Even though it's unlikely, complications can and do occur. Your best weapons include educating yourself about what your body is truly capable of and keeping a positive attitude. Keep in mind complications can occur anywhere, including at the hospital.

None of the information in this book should be taken as medical advice. While this guide intends to lead you through pregnancy and childbirth in a helpful, non-invasive way, sometimes medical assistance is required. Please don't hesitate to obtain such help.

Note on Genders

I use 'he' and 'she' interchangeably for the baby's gender. Some chapters will have boy babies, and some will have girl babies, and some may have both. You're encouraged to have babies of either sex (or both, if you like). The baby's gender certainly plays no role in your ability to give birth to him or her naturally.

References and Sources

I didn't write this book as a medical reference for professional childbirth attendants, such as doctors, midwives, or doulas. But if I presented a statement as a fact in this book, I've tried to provide a reference or source. I list the sources in the endnotes of each chapter and in the reference section at the end of the book.

Since I'm neither a legal researcher nor a medical professional, some of my sources may not appear valid to some people. But that's not really my point. You can always find a statistic or a study to back up a claim, however crazy or unrealistic the claim is. My goal was to find information that didn't ignore common sense.

For example, some women use castor oil to induce labor. Very few studies have been conducted to research the effects of castor oil on the mother and her baby. [1] Therefore, we have to rely on the experiences of individuals, which can vary, and draw our own conclusions.

With pregnancy and childbirth, I encourage you to use your common sense and your instincts, and the knowledge you have gathered along the way. It doesn't mean you shouldn't seek advice, but you have to weigh the information carefully.

Since you're educating yourself about natural childbirth, I trust you'll read other books on the subject. In fact, I encourage you to read as much as you need until you feel comfortable giving birth the way you want to.

---

[1] U.S. National Library of Medicine "Castor oil for induction of labour: not harmful, not helpful". Aust N ZJ Obstet Gynaecol, 49(5), 499-503. Retrieved from https://obgyn.onlinelibrary.wiley.com/doi/abs/10.1111/j.1479-828X.2009.01055.x

Chapter 1

About Natural Childbirth

In most highly developed nations, we have different options available for giving birth. In the United States, most women give birth in a hospital with a doctor present. But women may choose to give birth in a hospital with a certified nurse midwife in attendance. Midwives also attend births at freestanding birth centers and at the home of the mother. Last but not least, women can choose to give birth unassisted without having a medically trained attendant at the birth.

Unassisted births mostly happen at home. Sometimes women have an unplanned, unassisted birth if their labor progresses faster than they expected. For example, the baby may be born at home or on the way to the hospital or birth center.

The exact breakdown according to the Centers for Disease Control and Prevention is: "In 2010, 98.8 percent of all U.S. births occurred in hospitals. Among the 1.2 percent of out-of-hospital births, 67.0 percent were in a residence (home) and 28.0 percent were in a freestanding birthing center. Medical doctors attended the vast majority (86.3 percent) of hospital births in 2010, followed by certified nurse midwives (CNMs) (7.6 percent), and doctors of osteopathy (5.7 percent)."[1]

While there's a major difference between giving birth at the hospital and giving birth at home, women wanting to give birth naturally should focus more on the birth itself than the location or the attendant. It is certainly possible to have an unmedicated, natural childbirth in a hospital with a doctor in attendance. However, if you want to give birth naturally, you need to prepare for it.

From personal experience, I know that wanting to give birth without pain medication or other interventions does not guarantee a pleasant experience for you. You can increase your chances of having a natural birth by choosing supportive birth attendants. You must inform yourself about childbirth to make decisions during labor and birth.

When you give birth at a birth center or at home, the option of pain medication is usually not available to you. While I don't think this is the only reason you end up giving birth naturally, it certainly changes your mindset. Instead of a birth plan specifying you would prefer not to have anesthetics, you have already made a definite choice before labor begins.

As of today, there are no statistics available for unassisted births, partially because the trend is small, and partially because women giving birth unassisted rarely take part in data collection as is done in hospitals. However, my impression is that many women decide to have an unassisted birth only after having experienced one or more births in a different setting.

There are certainly freebirthers who chose an unassisted birth with their first child. The most widely known example is probably Laura Shanley, who gave birth to all her children unassisted.

You may not know anyone who gave birth unassisted, but it doesn't mean you're the only one. Most freebirthers only share their birth experience with close friends or on internet forums, where they can remain anonymous. Since many people are simply not supportive of unassisted childbirth, it's difficult to share those experiences with others. If you've given birth at home, I would certainly encourage you to let other women know that childbirth is not a scary but a wonderful experience. And maybe one day, all women will have faith in their own bodies again.

History of Childbirth

Although the physical act of giving birth has been the same for as long as humans have been around, there are still considerable differences in how women give birth, whether past or present. In biblical times, midwives were around to help women give birth. During those times, midwives were already recognized as a legitimate female profession.[2]

Midwives assisted women in childbirth, for which they would bring a birth stool. They believed it was beneficial to sit upright during birth. The birth stool had a hole in the middle, where the baby would fall through, to be caught by the midwife. However, only wealthy families could afford a midwife. Poor mothers had to make do with female relatives.

In the 1900s, women expected death and pain with childbirth. They viewed the pain in childbirth as punishment for the sins of Eve. It's no wonder childbirth was painful for those women, because of their expectations. If you expect a lot of pain, a hard labor and birth may be more likely, because of the mind-body connection. That being said, expecting a pain-free labor and birth doesn't guarantee you won't experience any pain.

In the 20th century, doctors gradually replaced midwives, even though previously men weren't allowed in the same room with a woman giving birth. After doctors started dominating the field of childbirth, midwives had to become licensed.

In England, the church was involved with licensing and required midwives to follow their religious ideas. They did this to conquer the fear of witchcraft, which was still prevalent. A midwife with questionable methods—methods not in line with church politics— would have lived in fear of being burned at the stake.

When doctors started monopolizing the field of childbirth, midwives became a minority and almost a thing of the past. In the 1940s and

1950s, most women gave birth in hospitals, except for the ones who lived in out-of-reach places. With the newly invented chloroform, labor was advertised as pain-free for all.[3]

With birth taking place at the hospital, many doctors increasingly used forceps and routine episiotomies just to get the baby out, mostly ignoring the natural process of childbirth. Only women living in rural areas would have their babies at home and most likely still have a natural childbirth by default.

In recent decades, the natural childbirth movement has made a comeback. As much as women demanded pain relief at the beginning of the 20th century, they now wanted to have their babies as nature intended. This also included a comeback for breastfeeding, which had been so widely replaced by formula.[4]

Midwifery in the United States

In the United States, there are different kinds of midwives today. Nurse-midwives work in hospitals. Their training and beliefs often closely mirror those of regular doctors. However, some nurse-midwives and virtually all direct-entry midwives work in the community or in the homes of mothers-to-be.

Direct-entry midwives study midwifery without prior education as a nurse. There are different types of direct-entry midwives, for example certified professional midwife, licensed midwife, and lay midwife. The difference in the title is the type of certification received, if any. Each state has different laws on how midwifery can be practiced. Where allowed, midwives will often form a birth center group. Many midwives attend homebirths, but this is not legal in every state.

We can count ourselves lucky to have these choices today. While they often interfere in the natural process of childbirth in many hospitals, at least those interventions are less likely to result in the death of the infant or the mother. When hospitals first became the setting for childbirth, many women died of infections, which were spread around at the hospital.[5]

Still, human beings wouldn't have made it this far if the act of childbirth required medical intervention. Most of the world does not get any, and yet women continue to have babies.

It's almost as if our bodies were meant to do so...

Childbirth in Different Cultures

Childbirth across the globe can differ in the location, the attendants, interventions used during birth, and even in the birthing position of the laboring woman. There are many differences in the treatment of the new mother and baby after the birth as well.

In 1900, almost all births occurred outside of hospitals, most of them at home.[6] Today, the opposite is true in the United States and many other countries. But giving birth in a hospital doesn't mean it has to a highly medicalized event.

In Sweden and Holland, which are both industrialized countries just like the United States, midwives help women give birth. In Holland, most babies are born at home. In Sweden, even though most of the births occur in hospitals, they don't encourage the use of epidurals. C-sections by choice are unheard of in both countries, and medical interventions are only used in emergencies.

In most countries, breastfeeding is encouraged. The United States is behind on this trend. In some hospitals, they even offer new mothers free formula samples for their babies. However, some hospitals and nursing staff are more supportive of breastfeeding than others. They may even offer the services of a lactation consultant for new mothers who need a little extra help.

In the United States, the traditional birthing position is for women to be on their backs with their shoulders propped up, forcing them to work against gravity to birth their babies. Most of the rest of the world chooses more suitable birthing positions, such as squatting, kneeling, standing, and sometimes even hanging. When it comes to natural childbirth, we still have much to learn from other cultures.

There are still societies in which giving birth unassisted is natural, even today. In some cultures, they consider this the ideal way to have a baby. While a pregnant woman in the United States seems to require extra medical care for nine months and medical attendants and equipment in order to give birth, women in those societies often give birth without any help at all.

Examples of such societies are the !Kung, San Bushmen, and Bariba. For all three cultures, giving birth alone is an ideal worth striving for.[7] Many first-time mothers don't achieve this goal, but unassisted births still account for at least half of all births.

!Kung girls are encouraged to watch a woman give birth, to help them face their fears. They're expected to face the pain of childbirth with courage. This presents a stark contrast to childbirth in the United States, where medical attendants encourage epidurals. In modern societies, even women who don't plan on receiving pain relief in the form of medications still use special techniques to cope with the pain of labor and childbirth, such as relaxation, breathing techniques, counter pressure, massage, and visualization.

!Kung women give birth alone by going into the bushes. They bury their placenta before returning to the village with their newborn baby. The burying of the placenta can happen in the United States as well, more often by women giving birth at home. For the African tribes, burying the placenta has a higher meaning. They believe the placenta belongs to Mother Earth, and therefore, it has to be returned.

Another major difference between a tribal woman and her American counterpart is the tribal woman is active throughout her pregnancy. She must fulfill her regular duties without complaint. Pregnant women in industrialized countries often use their pregnancy as a time to overeat and put their feet up. Obviously, staying active is the better choice, and it will prevent both the woman and her baby from gaining too much weight.

We don't have to give birth exactly the same way those tribal women do, but reading about them can be inspiring. Their faith in the natural process of pregnancy and childbirth is encouraging. And since we have even more information and resources at our disposal, we should be able to give birth just as easily as they do.

Why Childbirth Is Medically Supervised

Unfortunately, hospitals, doctors, and the drug industry all benefit from medical interventions. It takes less time to perform a C-section than it does to be present for an entire natural labor and birth. Therefore, scheduled C-sections may have become too popular, partly because they help doctors see more patients in less time.

When a woman in labor gets admitted to the hospital, she will most likely not even see her doctor until she is ready to have her baby. In the meantime, she is being cared for by other nursing staff. This makes me wonder why we spend so much time on finding the right doctor. In the end, you'll probably spend more time with the nurses at your hospital than with your doctor, even if you add up all your prenatal visits prior to giving birth.

Giving birth at the hospital can be expensive. And while money isn't the only reason labor and childbirth are medically supervised, it may be the predominant one. The hospital earns more money when more resources are needed, whether it's special equipment or highly trained staff. For example, a fetal monitoring system and an on-call anesthesiologist increase the cost of birth and the bottom line of the hospital.

Some medical procedures reduce the operating costs of the hospital, either by making it less expensive for the hospital or more efficient for the staff. Such an example would be the use of the fetal monitoring system.

And at first glance, it allows labor to progress efficiently. One nurse can monitor several fetal monitors without being physically present with the laboring women. However, it doesn't mean using fetal monitoring is a good thing (more on this topic later). In comparison, most midwives rely on the use of a Doppler instead, but this requires a more active, personal, and hands-on approach.

Another reason childbirth "requires" a lot of interventions is the rise of lawsuits. Unfortunately, doctors have to intervene whenever the slightest complication demands it, to avoid getting sued. Sadly enough, if complications arise, doctors get sued over the interventions they didn't perform and not because they performed too many interventions.

Therefore, it is legally safest for them to use as many interventions as possible. If a case goes to court, then they can say they've tried everything. Having to worry about malpractice lawsuits is not helpful for doctors who want to make good decisions. Sometimes, what's best for the patient is not what the doctor learned in medical school.

Being afraid of lawsuits doesn't just affect the way doctors practice medicine. Doctors have to carry expensive malpractice insurance, which increases already high health-care costs. Even if they don't use any medical equipment in the hospital, you still have to pay more for giving birth there than for a birth at home or at a birth center.

Medical doctors who believe in the woman's ability to give birth still exist today. If you can find one, he or she can help you have a great natural birth. Unfortunately, most doctors are trained for emergencies, and they really believe childbirth is dangerous if it isn't medically supervised.

Speaking in defense of doctors, I believe almost all of them honestly think they're helping. They don't intervene intending to sabotage labor, even though that's likely a result. They really want to help. As a general rule, even the best intentions do not make medical interventions useful in childbirth.

While most doctors obviously don't support unassisted childbirth, you may find more midwives who are open to the idea. As a group, midwives have been quiet about unassisted childbirth. They know women can have babies on their own. In fact, it's their job to assist them with giving birth without medical interventions. But while most midwives certainly realize women can give birth on their own, they also depend on women using their services.

I'm thankful for the existence of modern medicine. Modern medicine can save lives when they would otherwise be lost, especially in an emergency. However, Walter Cronkite may have said it best: "America's health care system is neither healthy, caring, nor a system."

If we were all healthy, we wouldn't need hospitals, doctors, and prescription drugs as much as we do, would we? It's in the medical community's best interest that we remain ignorant about our own body and its self-healing abilities. Childbirth and pregnancy are just one of the many things hospitals and doctors can profit on.

We all need to take charge of our own health and well-being. And giving birth on your own is something almost all women are naturally capable of.

The Dangers of Interventions

Childbirth is a natural process, just as much as digestion. Many women fear they won't know what to do, especially if they've never had a baby before. But you don't need anyone to tell you when to push, just as you don't need anyone to tell you when to have a bowel movement. Your body will let you know. Even if you did nothing at all, your body will eventually give birth, whether you want to or not.

When modern medicine is involved in childbirth, there can be many interventions, most of them at the hospital. All interventions have side effects, probably even more than the ones I've listed in these pages. Therefore, it's almost always better to let nature do its job without interfering.

You can find literature defending the use of some or all these interventions, and you can find studies emphasizing their harmful consequences. In the end, you'll need to decide for yourself what you're willing to put up with and where you draw the line.

Remember, it's your body, and it's your baby.

The Vaginal Exam

During pregnancy and labor, standard medical care includes several vaginal exams. Even though a vaginal exam may not seem like a big deal, it can actually be harmful.

For one, vaginal exams increase the risk of an infection. If you tried to examine your own cervix (difficult but possible), you're unlikely to cause an infection, unless you introduce foreign objects.

A doctor or midwife can't know exactly what a vaginal exam feels like to you. It's even possible for them to rupture your membranes accidentally (or, more worrisome, on purpose against your will). Spotting and cramping after a vaginal exam is common. You may not feel any pain during a vaginal exam, but it can be very uncomfortable.

One purpose of vaginal exams is to check dilation and effacement at the end of your pregnancy. However, neither can accurately predict when labor is going to start. During labor, the amount of dilation can give a woman false hope her baby will be there soon. Conversely, it could make the doctors think labor is not progressing fast enough. This is because the dilation of your cervix can happen fast or slowly. Nobody knows how long it will take to go from 3 centimeters to 10. It could take an hour, or it could take several weeks.

According to the New Zealand College of Midwives, the vaginal exam should be used sparingly: "[The vaginal exam] may be an unnecessary intervention if used routinely and as part of standardised labour care. Vaginal examination should be used judiciously when there is a need for more information that cannot be gained from observing the various external aspects of labour."[8]

If you choose to give birth with a midwife, she may support this point of view. Often, under the midwifery model of care, you'll undergo fewer examinations during pregnancy and labor. Many midwives recognize it's best to interfere as little as possible to ensure a safe, natural birth.

IV Fluids

Most hospital births require the use of an IV as standard procedure for laboring women. In theory, an IV sounds like a good idea to give you much-needed fluids. The question is: do you really need fluids through a tube?

The fluids from the IV nourish your body, but you may still feel hungry and thirsty. However, in most hospitals, you're not allowed to eat or drink during labor. This makes no sense. It deprives the body of nourishment, and therefore, the laboring woman may run out of energy before her baby is born, which often leads to additional interventions.[9]

IV fluids can wreak havoc in your body. They dilute your blood stream unnaturally, which can decrease the concentration of oxytocin and other hormones your body needs to labor efficiently. When you're attached to an IV, you can't walk around easily. Finally, there is always a risk of infection at the site of the IV, which is usually on your hand or wrist.

An article published by the Journal of Perinatal Education has this to say about IVs: "With no evidence that their routine use is beneficial, a small but consistent body of evidence that they can cause harm, and important questions unanswered, a change in practice is long overdue."[10] Using IVs routinely is not a good idea, yet it continues to be common practice.

Pitocin and Induction of Labor

Doctors often administer Pitocin to induce labor. Most often, labor is induced by 41 weeks, or 42 weeks at the latest. Practitioners even induce before the due date, because it's convenient either for the doctor or the woman.

However, inducing labor is always risky. If labor hasn't started naturally, it means your baby is not ready to be born. If your baby was ready, labor would begin on its own.

Doctors may induce labor when they suspect a large baby, because they're worried it may not fit through the birth canal. The actual likelihood of it happening is close to zero. I couldn't find any statistics describing the number of women whose pelvis was too small to give birth to their baby. And yet, many doctors offer precisely this argument as a reason for a C-section.

Besides, ultrasounds often over- or underestimate the size of the baby. Medical professionals don't take into consideration how much room your body can make for your baby. For example, a simple change in position (from lying down to squatting) widens your pelvis considerably, allowing for the safe passage of your baby.

Certain drugs can speed up labor if labor is not progressing or not progressing fast enough, according to your provider's time clock. These drugs will be administered through an IV and can cause additional problems.

Any medication entering your system through the IV will affect your baby, too, although the medical community declares all those drugs to be safe. Your baby will receive some of everything they give you, either through the placenta or through the breastmilk.

"Lamaze International recommends that a woman allows her body to go into labor on its own, unless there is a true medical reason to induce. Allowing labor to start on its own reduces the possibility of complications, including a vacuum or forceps-assisted birth, fetal heart rate changes, babies with low birth weight or jaundice, and cesarean surgery. Studies consistently show that inducing labor almost doubles a woman's chance of having cesarean surgery."[11]

The risks of inductions outweigh the benefits in most cases. Just because a woman has gone past her due date or is tired of being pregnant is not a reason to induce labor. A legitimate reason to induce would be a health problem in the mother or the baby that compromises the well-being of either of them.

Fetal Monitoring

One of the biggest problems in hospitals is the routine use of fetal monitoring. Whenever hospital staff administers Pitocin or another labor-inducing drug (and often even when they don't), they require the laboring woman to be attached to a fetal monitor. The fetal monitor continuously records the baby's heart rate and the mother's contractions, but the mother can't leave the hospital bed. If the baby shows any unfavorable reactions to the contractions, this is taken to be a sign of fetal distress. Whenever such fetal distress is diagnosed and birth is not imminent, more interference is required.

Maybe it's time to stop and reconsider the problem. If labor hadn't been induced in the first place, the baby may not be distressed at being kicked out early. Fetal monitoring systems regularly diagnose fetal distress in error. As a result, many C-sections are performed unnecessarily.

Fetal monitoring can take place in two different ways, externally and internally. For external monitoring, the laboring woman wears a belt around her belly, which records her contractions and the fetal heart rate. Internal monitoring can only be done after the water has been broken (usually by a doctor). The doctor then attaches an electrode to the baby's head to measure his vitals.

Here's what Natural Motherhood has to say about fetal monitoring: "The profound message of the external and internal fetal monitors is that your body is so defective and in danger from potential malfunction that it is necessary to apply a special machine to more exactly monitor your baby to protect him from potential harm caused by you. And that even justifies screwing an electrode in your baby's head without the benefit of pain medication if need be!"[12]

During a natural labor and birth, your body's contractions will not harm your baby. Therefore, it shouldn't be necessary to monitor your baby this way. Unfortunately, with an induction, the contractions are not natural anymore. This is another reason to avoid having labor jump-started for you.

Breaking the Water Artificially

At the hospital, the staff will have expectations for your labor you may not meet. After checking in, the staff expects women to give birth within 12 to 24 hours. If labor isn't progressing fast enough according to hospital protocols, the doctor or midwife may decide to break your bag of waters. During an amniotomy (breaking of the waters), the doctor or midwife will manually insert their finger into your cervix and rupture your membranes.

Breaking the waters is supposed to speed up labor, but studies have found it has not done so verifiably. A Cochrane review of available studies concluded: "Evidence does not support routinely breaking the waters for women in normally progressing spontaneous labour or where labours have become prolonged. [...] Routine amniotomy is not recommended as part of standard labour management and care."[13]

Your contractions can become stronger after the bag of waters has been forcibly broken. The baby can be harmed as well, because now his head is not protected as he moves through the birth canal. Without the bag of waters, the cushion is gone for the woman, which can make labor more painful. This increases the likelihood for administering additional pain relief.

Breaking the water can even lead to prolapse of the umbilical cord, which can be life threatening to the baby. According to an article in Midwifery Today, "1 cord prolapse results from every 300 amniotomies".[14]

Cord prolapse describes a situation in which the umbilical cord descends into the vagina prematurely before the baby's head. This means during contractions and pushing, the baby's circulation is cut off, as pressure is being put onto the cord. This can lead to fetal brain damage or death. The only thing that can save your baby now is an immediate C-section.

According to childbirth educator Henci Goer, "Cord prolapse is most likely when membranes are ruptured early in labor when the head is still high, as would happen with inductions."[15]

Pain Relief

Pain is bad and should be avoided at all costs, right? Not quite. When you receive pain relief during labor, you're actually being deprived emotionally. It seems counterintuitive at first.

After nine months of being pregnant and several hours of being in labor, you expect and deserve the climax of giving birth. When you're denied the climax of birth, it can take you longer to bond with your baby, and you may feel sad, missing something without knowing what that is.[16]

As much as we all want to avoid pain, labor pains are truly different. During labor, the pain increases gradually as the contractions get stronger. And just when you think you can't handle it anymore, it's time to have your baby. As soon as the baby is born, the pain vanishes. Instead, you experience euphoria. It's an amazing feeling to give birth and hold your newborn baby in your arms. Personally, I found the pain of labor and birth excruciating towards the end. Yet, I would have willingly given birth again a few seconds after each of my babies was born. The only exception was my first birth where I couldn't feel anything with the epidural. That's how powerful the pain and the resulting climax can be.

You could compare labor and childbirth to a roller-coaster ride. If you're drugged up during either, you won't realize when the ride is over. As a result, your body has a hard time adjusting to what's going on. Besides taking away most sensations, epidurals can cause serious harm. After all, the anesthesiologist is inserting a needle into your spine. Naturally, this procedure comes with risks, and those should never be taken lightly.

In addition to the potential side effects, administering pain relief results in the loss of control for the laboring woman. For a first-time mother, not knowing what to expect can make it worse. Epidurals sometimes don't work at all, but some women get so numb they can't feel anything. In the latter case, you'd have to rely on doctors and nurses to tell you when to push. But how would they know what your body needs you to do?

Positioning

Your position during labor is often another choice you don't get to make for yourself at the hospital. Laboring on your back is probably the worst way to have your baby, but unfortunately, it has become the standard. In this position, you're birthing your baby against the forces of gravity. It also decreases your flexibility. Your pelvis and cervix can widen considerably to make room for your baby's head, but not while you're on your back.

The results of giving birth while lying on your back vary, but they can include tearing and failure to progress. This position is only good for the birth attendants, because it allows them to see what's going on. They can see the baby crowning, and they can "catch" him or her. I find it somewhat ironic that modern medicine warns you to stay off your back during the second and third trimester, but then expects you to give birth in that same position.

The good news is things are changing. Even the World Health Organization has good things to say about upright positioning during labor and birth: "Giving birth in an upright position appears to be associated with several benefits, including reduction in the duration of the second stage of labour."[17]

Episiotomy

When labor is not progressing and your baby is not moving down the birth canal as expected, your doctor may perform an episiotomy to get the baby out. An episiotomy can often be avoided when a more favorable birthing position is chosen. After an episiotomy is performed, you have to get stitches, and there's no chance of an intact perineum. Many medical professionals still believe episiotomies prevent severe tearing, even though studies show the opposite is true.[18]

Vacuum and Forceps

A doctor may resort to an episiotomy if the baby needs to be born quickly, if the baby is large, or to use forceps or a vacuum. Forceps look like salad tongs and are used to help pull the baby out, while you're pushing during a contraction. A vacuum looks like a plunger. It's attached to the baby's head, and the pressure difference of the air is used to help extract the baby.

Forceps require an episiotomy, but for a vacuum extraction an episiotomy may not be necessary. Of course, both methods come with their own sets of risks. The most serious one is intracranial hemorrhage of the newborn.

According to the American Journal of Epidemiology "Intracranial hemorrhage was higher among infants delivered by vacuum extraction, forceps, or cesarean section (after onset of labor only) than among infants delivered vaginally without instrumentation."[19] Either intervention will make this birth unpleasant for you and more painful.

Fortunately, the use of both forceps and vacuum can often be completely avoided by repositioning the laboring woman. Switching to a different position, such as squatting or standing, will often be enough to encourage the descent of the baby. And if a woman was left alone to labor, she would probably not choose to labor on her back. Instincts would have her move around and switch positions. What makes moving around more difficult (or even impossible) is continuous fetal monitoring, an IV, and an epidural.

C-Section

The ultimate intervention is probably a C-section. Unfortunately, C-sections are often performed even when they're medically unnecessary. For lack of a better reason, doctors may cite fetal distress or a large baby.

Your body was not so poorly designed that your baby would be too big to be born vaginally. Back when women wore corsets, this may have been a problem, because the corsets actually changed the shape of their pelvis. However, I don't think corsets are worn much at all anymore, at least not in the United States.

Yet, C-sections are on the rise, and there are even women who chose them over a vaginal birth. In some countries, such as Brazil and Taiwan, a C-section is the fashionable way to have a baby, because it allows the woman to keep an intact vagina.[20]

But a C-section is major abdominal surgery, and it's risky. Not only are you at risk because of anesthesia but because of the procedure itself. Your baby is at risk, too. In an interview for National Healthy Mothers, Healthy Babies Coalition, Dr. Sakala stated a "C-section can also cause other problems for a baby, who may be cut (usually minor) during surgery. Cesarean-born babies are also more likely to have breathing problems around the time of birth and to experience asthma in childhood and adulthood."[21]

Unfortunately, C-sections are still too common, as described by the vital statistics report: "In 2010, the cesarean delivery rate was 32.8 percent of all births, down from 32.9 percent in 2009 (Table 21). This is the first decrease in the overall cesarean delivery rate since 1996."[22] The decrease of 0.1% is hardly worth noting, but at least the rate of C-sections isn't increasing. Many people, myself included, find it hard to believe a third of all births truly require a C-section. There's obviously something wrong with our medical system.

An additional problem with having a C-section is the negative psychological effects of such a birth on the mother. If you've ever spoken to someone who ended up with a C-section, you know they don't cherish their birth experience at all. In fact, they may even doubt their own ability to give birth naturally the next time around.

Suctioning Baby's Nose and Mouth

The interventions don't end when your baby is born. After the birth, medical procedures will focus on your newborn baby instead of on you. And since modern practitioners don't believe labor or childbirth can happen naturally without interference, they also don't think your baby will be fine on her own.

Therefore, as soon as your baby is born, medical staff will suction his nose and mouth and vigorously rub his back to ensure he breathes. While most healthy babies start breathing immediately when they're exposed to oxygen, doctors and midwives routinely suction babies, anyway. While this may not sound harmful to your baby, it is (more on this in the chapter on childbirth). In short, suctioning interferes with the birthing process. Your baby should be held in loving arms (yours or your partner's) after birth and not be subjected to such rough handling.

Placenta and Umbilical Cord

After the birth of your baby, doctors and midwives are concerned with the birth of your placenta. Naturally, this can take some time. At the hospital, the medical staff expect the placenta within minutes of giving birth. Otherwise, they will tug on it and/or administer drugs (such as Pitocin) to make your uterus contract.

If doctors were not so quick to separate mother and baby, the placenta would make its appearance with little delay. When you nurse your baby, your uterus receives oxytocin, making it contract, which helps your body birth the placenta.

Besides hurrying the placenta, hospital staff may be quick to cut the cord. Cutting the cord while it's still pulsating robs your baby of a lot of blood he could have used, because the blood from the placenta provides valuable oxygen and nutrients. By the way, banking the cord blood for future use also deprives your baby of the blood he needs now.

Taking Measurements

While the medical staff is concentrating on the birth of your placenta, your baby is usually taken away from you. After the traumatic birth (from the baby's point of view), your baby doesn't even get to be in your arms where you can comfort him. For a healthy baby and mother, there is no medical need to separate mother and child after birth. Measuring and weighing the baby should wait.

Unfortunately, doctors and nurses have to satisfy hospital protocols. Midwives at homebirths are usually much more understanding of the need to bond. They will check your baby's heart rate while you're holding her, and they will often wait with measuring and weighing until later. Unfortunately, by the time the mother finally gets to hold her new baby at the hospital, he will be all swaddled up. This does not allow for skin-to-skin contact, which is so important for newborn babies and new mothers.

Eye Ointment and Vitamin K Shot

After examining your baby, doctors and nurses will administer treatments. They treat all babies for infections they don't have, even the ones who were born perfectly healthy.

For example, the eye ointment is supposed to protect the baby's eyes from sexually transmitted diseases the mother might have. This procedure is done routinely, even though mothers are routinely tested for those same diseases during pregnancy. If your test for STDs during pregnancy comes back negative, the eye ointment will still be administered to your baby. It's bizarre and illogical.

At the hospital, your baby will receive a Vitamin K shot. The shot can lead to complications[23]. The Vitamin K administered is many times the amount an infant needs. The shot includes other unpronounceable ingredients we inject into his little system, too.

Here is another noteworthy point: babies are more or less universally born with low Vitamin K levels. Should it then really be considered a deficiency state, when in fact, there might be a reason for it we just don't know about yet?

Besides the potential physical side effects, both the eye ointment and the Vitamin K shot significantly interfere with bonding. The eye ointment blurs your baby's vision, preventing him from focusing on your face. The Vitamin K shot, in addition to all the other administrations, wears your baby out. He may not even have the energy to latch on properly afterwards, interfering with breastfeeding.

Even though babies can't talk, they're aware of their surroundings. Therefore, let's show our babies we love them from the moment they're born, by protecting them from harmful interventions and keeping them in our arms.

While I dedicated a sizeable portion of this chapter talking about the harm of interventions, there's much more to be said on the subject. For the readers who still need to be convinced why natural childbirth is the best way, I encourage you to read Laura Shanley's book called "Unassisted Childbirth".

The Use of Medical Interventions

You may believe medical interventions are problematic, but they do have their place. When something goes wrong, modern medicine can potentially do a world of good. Some women and babies are only here today because the mother had a C-section. Similarly, some women may have an ectopic pregnancy and would have never found out about it if it hadn't been for an ultrasound.

The fundamental problem with interventions is they're not used as judiciously as they should be. Does every pregnant woman require an ultrasound? Does every woman in labor require frequent vaginal exams or fetal monitoring or an IV? Common sense and statistics will tell you most women give birth to healthy babies without a problem.

There's a time and a place for medical help. If you're ever in doubt, please seek medical assistance. Your health and that of your baby are always the primary considerations during pregnancy and childbirth.

You also have to accept life doesn't come without risks. Interventions are risky, but things could go wrong without them. It's up to you to decide which of the options presents the greater risk, but nobody can guarantee a perfect outcome either way.

On a positive note, your odds are pretty good everything will be fine. Once you have educated yourself and made your choices about childbirth and pregnancy, you can sit back and relax and trust in the process.

Your Rights as a Patient

Some interventions are annoying, but others seem downright scary. Fortunately, you may refuse any and all procedures the doctor requires. Technically, nobody can be forced into receiving medical treatment at the hospital. But if you were in a critical medical condition and unable to talk, doctors would certainly do everything in their power to save your life.

Unfortunately, hospital staff members don't always ask for your consent for many procedures performed during labor and childbirth. For example, you probably won't have the option to refuse an IV or fetal monitoring. And even if you don't consent to certain procedures, you might be bullied, coerced, or otherwise forced into complying. In extreme cases, doctors have even obtained court orders or involved Child Protective Services. This has gone so far that the term "birth rape" was coined to describe these situations.

As scary as all of this sounds, even if you go to the hospital to give birth, you may still refuse some or all of the treatments. It's your right. However, one reason women give birth at home is they don't think their wishes will be honored at the hospital.

The bottom line is: it's your body. You have the right to protect yourself. And once your baby is born, it's your job to keep him from harm as well.

Choosing Your Midwife

Skip this section if you already have your heart set on an unassisted birth. But some women like to hire a midwife as a backup for their planned homebirth, and there's nothing wrong with that.

Most women who give birth at home do so with a midwife in attendance. A midwife-attended homebirth is also often the stepping stone for an unassisted homebirth with a later pregnancy. The right midwife can be a very comforting presence. For the best possible birth experience, choose your midwife carefully.

During early pregnancy is a good time to meet with different care providers to find one you click with. Depending on where you live, you may not have a lot of options available to you. There may only be one or a couple of midwives who accept patients. Sometimes you have to drive quite a distance to visit with your midwife for prenatal appointments.

Since you want to give birth at home, it's important to make the distinction in your search for midwives, because you can find licensed midwives that work at doctor's offices and in hospitals, too. They may give you the same level of care, but they won't be coming to your home for the birth.

When you hire a midwife, you may be able to give birth at the birth center instead of at your home. You can take your time in deciding whether that's a good choice for you or not. If your midwife offers both options, she probably won't require you to pick one or the other until you're closer to your due date.

Many midwives practice in small groups to reduce the number of night shifts they have to work. In that case, you probably won't get to pick which midwife will be at your birth. Therefore, get to know all the midwives during your pregnancy to help you establish a bond with each of them.

Even though a homebirth midwife is unlikely to intervene unnecessarily, ask where she stands on the following topics before procuring her services:

- Induction of labor
- Assisted birth (forceps or vacuum)
- Allowing time for the placenta to arrive
- Post-term pregnancy
- Risk factors that require her to refer you to an obstetrician
- Ability to delay or skip newborn procedures
- Option to drink and eat during labor
- Option to delay or skip certain prenatal tests
- Option to be hands-off during the birth

You don't have to ask your midwife all the questions at once. But if you really want your midwife to be hands-off during the birth, then it's important to find out if that even works for her before you hire her.

Similarly, if you plan on delaying or skipping certain prenatal tests, it might be a good idea to find out if she will allow this under her care. It might not be a big deal to skip an ultrasound, but her license requirements may not let you get out of other tests, including the glucose tolerance test and the Group Beta Strep test.

Some midwives work together with an obstetrician who they refer patients to, when necessary. In this case, you can have a natural birth even if you end up having your baby in the hospital because of unforeseen circumstances. Other midwives don't have any other option but to drop you from their care when it becomes too risky. For example, your midwife might not attend your homebirth if you're diagnosed with gestational diabetes or high blood pressure. It's important to understand ahead of time what will happen in that case.

While you always have the option to give birth at home unassisted, it might not be the best solution if you have medical issues. Of course, sometimes it's also possible your midwife can't be your provider for legal reasons, even though it would be safe for you and your baby to have a homebirth. For example, your midwife will most likely not be able to attend your birth if you go past 42 or 43 weeks of pregnancy.

Having Students at Your Birth

Since people aren't born midwives but have to train to become one, it's only logical they have to attend births as a student midwife to learn the ropes. As the star of the show, you should have a say in the decision to include students at your birth.

Some midwives don't mention that there may be students, and it just happens. If you like the students or don't mind their presence, then that's okay. However, if you'd rather not have them at your birth, you should feel comfortable enough to make your opinion known.

When I was under the care of a midwife, she told me I could decide who was present at my birth. If I didn't like someone (unless it was one of midwives), then that person wouldn't be at my birth. It sounds simple, but let it sink in a bit, because this is very profound: **It's your birth, and you get to decide who will attend.** You also get to decide who isn't welcome, even if it hurts someone's feelings for being excluded.

Just be aware, there's a decent chance your midwife won't show up alone. She may bring an assistant, a nurse, another midwife, or a student midwife.

Birth Center vs. Homebirth

When you seek midwifery care, you may choose to give birth at a birth center or at home. You don't have to decide which option is right for you until you get closer to your due date. But at some point, you need to weigh your options.

Birth centers have certain advantages. For example, they usually have a very nice, enormous bathtub for you to labor and give birth in. The birth center may be more centrally located than your home, in case you need emergency assistance. And last but not least, birth centers are usually well stocked with everything you need during labor and birth.

The downside to going to a birth center is you have to get in the car while you're in labor. Since you have to travel to give birth, you may also end up going there sooner than necessary. Most birth centers allow you to stay for several hours after the birth (or until the next morning), but then you have to get in the car again, this time with your newborn baby.

Personally, I preferred giving birth at home because I didn't have to go anywhere. I didn't have to get dressed. I didn't have to sit in an uncomfortable car seat during contractions. And after the birth, I could just rest with my newborn without having to get presentable enough to drive home.

If you or your significant other feel better about the birth center because of its proximity to a hospital, it might still be the right choice for you. If you just want to have a water birth, I recommend looking into purchasing or renting a birth pool. Your midwife can probably help you find one in your area, too.

If you currently don't live in a comfortable home or have to share housing with other people you'd rather not invite to your birth, a birth center might be a good option for you. Birth centers are usually very inviting and private. It certainly doesn't hurt to tour the place during one of your prenatal appointments.

Benefits of Unassisted Childbirth

Having a great childbirth experience is extremely important to the beginning of your parenting journey. Obviously, you can still form an attachment to your baby if you have to have a C-section and cannot breastfeed. However, it may take more time to fall in love with your baby. Giving birth naturally, while having all your wits about you, will help you form this bond immediately after birth.

A less-than-ideal birth may leave you feeling unsatisfied or even miserable. It can take weeks, months, or even years to make your peace with it. If you're not in charge of your birth experience, things may not turn out the way you planned.

Mothers who don't experience birth the way they wanted to are more likely to suffer from postpartum depression. A study done at the department of psychology by the Missouri Western State University had the following findings about this phenomenon: "The incidence and severity of postpartum depression has been found to be related to the place and type of delivery, the perceived level of control over the birth experience, and the satisfaction level. The home birth group was found to have the lowest rate of depression, have felt the most control over their birth experience, and were the most satisfied."[24]

It's possible an unassisted birth group would have even lower rates of depression than the homebirth group. However, unassisted births make up a tiny percentage of all births, and therefore, not much research has been done on them.

The study noted the satisfaction level of women who had homebirths was higher than that of women who had hospital births. Homebirthers also had more control over their experience. Could it be the level of satisfaction was higher *because* the women had more control over their experience? I bet so.

According to Christiane Northrup, M.D., "the connection between overuse of intervention and postpartum depression is enormous. If women experienced the ecstasy of birth, they would have the high that would get them through the hormonal changes of the next week."[25]

There are many reasons women choose to give birth unassisted. While you may have a lack of other homebirth options (midwife-attended homebirths are not legal in every state), you may choose unassisted childbirth for one or more of these reasons:

- Take control of your birth
- Limit or eliminate interventions
- Bond with your baby
- Connect with other family members
- Have a stress-free birth
- Support breastfeeding
- Choose the gentle(st) way to give birth

Preparing for an Unassisted Birth

Once you decide to give birth unassisted, the next step is to prepare for your birth. But before I discuss pregnancy and childbirth in more detail, I'd like to help you address any fears you may harbor about doing it all on your own.

Everyone is afraid sometimes. Being afraid is a natural reaction to real danger, and it can be useful. If you've never given birth before, you may be afraid because childbirth is unknown to you. Women who have watched other women give birth rarely harbor the same fears about childbirth. And while you may not have the option of attending an actual birth, you can definitely watch a video of one.

You may have created a scary picture of childbirth in your head. It could be a movie you've seen or a story you've read or heard about. And whether you're afraid of childbirth because it's a big unknown, or whether you're harboring specific fears, you must face your fears before you can conquer them.

Fear of the Unknown

I'm not a psychologist, nor do I have any special knowledge on the subject, but I understand being afraid can stop many people from doing what they really want to do. This includes being afraid of change and being afraid of the unknown. Many people won't even quit a job they despise, because they're afraid of the changes this will bring about.

If the thought of an unassisted birth gives you an uneasy feeling, then you need to dig a little deeper. The best way to get over any fears you may have is to pinpoint them.

My oldest daughter is afraid of many things, probably because she has a great imagination. One day (she was seven years old at the time), she cried, because she was afraid a fire might break out in her room. She has never been in a fire, and this incident seemed to happen out of the blue. My husband got her to focus by asking her what she would do if there really was a fire in her room. Our daughter said she would climb out the window. And after finding that solution, she stopped being afraid. Fortunately, imagining how to conquer a scary scenario is only one of many ways to handle your fear.

Conquering your fear becomes more difficult when you're dealing with a feeling of general uneasiness. What exactly is causing it? Doing something new can be scary, but you can handle it. Next time you feel apprehensive, you need to find out what you're afraid of by picturing the scenario.

If you've never given birth before, find some positive birth videos to watch. Watching a woman give birth naturally should restore your confidence and replace vague fears with actual information. Besides preparing you, it will help you ask the right questions. For example, what exactly happens first during childbirth, and what do you need to do?

You can get in touch with other women who have done what you're planning to do. Even if you don't know anyone personally, there are several online forums with women who are supportive of unassisted childbirth. Either they have done it, or they want to do it. At the time of this writing, you can find several unassisted childbirth groups on Facebook.

Conquer Your Fears Step by Step

Once you know what to expect, you may have other concerns. For each fear, go through the following steps:

1. Define what exactly you're afraid of.
2. Picture the scary scenario.
3. What would you do if it actually happened?
4. Find out how likely it is to happen.
5. Research how to prevent it from happening.
6. Decide how you want to prepare for that eventuality.

Example: You're afraid of too much bleeding after birth.

1. What are you afraid of? You're afraid of having a postpartum hemorrhage.

2. Picture the scary scenario: Postpartum hemorrhage involves an enormous amount of blood loss (over 500 ml or 2 cups within 24 hours of giving birth). Besides experiencing blood loss, you may feel dizzy or become unconscious.

3. What would you do if it actually happened? Should you experience postpartum hemorrhage, you could first try uterine massage to stimulate uterine contractions. If uterine massage doesn't work, medication is next. At the hospital, it would be oxytocin. At home, you can try herbs such as Arnica montana or Bellis perennis.[26] Some women chew on their placenta at the first sign of a hemorrhage. Finally, you can call an ambulance. (There's more information on what to do during a postpartum hemorrhage in the chapter on childbirth.)

4. How likely is it to happen? Postpartum hemorrhage is not a problem with 95% of all births. However, it's more likely when giving birth to multiples, when giving birth to a large baby, when laboring under Pitocin, after having a prolonged labor, or after having had more than five full-term pregnancies.[27]

5. How can you prevent postpartum hemorrhage? There are things you can do to prevent postpartum hemorrhage. During pregnancy, keep your iron levels up (more about anemia in a later chapter). During the second stage of labor, never pull on the umbilical cord. Instead, the placenta should be birthed naturally.[28] To encourage the placenta, it may help to breastfeed your newborn immediately after birth. Having an empty bladder will help your uterus contract. Therefore, you need to use the bathroom frequently during labor and afterwards.

6. How can you prepare for a postpartum hemorrhage? You can purchase specific herbs to have on hand, in case you need them. You can mentally prepare yourself to chew on the placenta to stop the bleeding. Finally, educate yourself about supplementation during pregnancy to reduce the likelihood of postpartum hemorrhage.

As you prepare for an unassisted birth, the most important advice anyone can give you is to have faith in yourself and your body. You can really do this, just as so many others have done before you. Feeling nervous ahead of time is natural, but ignoring your fears is not the answer.

What If Something Goes Wrong?

Unfortunately, it's easy to blame other people or circumstances when something goes wrong. For example, the doctor didn't prescribe antibiotics when he should have, or I'm overweight because my parents fed me junk food as a child. While both statements may be true, we still need to accept responsibility for our own health and the health of our children today.

It can be unsettling to be fully responsible for yourself and your baby during pregnancy. It's a lot easier to go to your prenatal appointments, as you have been told to do, and then report to the hospital for the birth. But in the end, even if you don't realize it, you're still responsible for yourself and your baby.

Even if doctors are there to assist you, they can't make you healthy. Receiving regular prenatal care doesn't make you healthy. Keeping up healthy habits during your pregnancy, such as eating right, exercising, and going outside regularly will help you and your baby stay healthy.

Back to the problem: what if something goes wrong? You've probably heard from someone who had a stillborn baby or a premature labor where the baby didn't survive. First, you need to realize that while there's always a possibility this may happen to you, the chances of it really happening are quite slim.

Besides, whether your baby is stillborn at home or at the hospital doesn't change the devastating and traumatic nature of such an event. Sometimes, being at a hospital can change the outcome. But sometimes, the baby dies in utero, and the birth itself is not the cause of the baby's death at all.

I don't wish a stillborn baby on anyone, and I can't imagine how hard it would be to suffer through. However, in view of an unassisted birth, this possibility may not be a big factor in your decision. While complications can arise during a homebirth, they are more likely in a hospital setting because of the way the natural process of birth is interfered with.

Giving birth unassisted is not child neglect. However, it means you need to take responsibility. And while you should certainly educate yourself about potential complications, you really don't need to worry too much about them. If fears like this held you back every day, you wouldn't drive a car (many more people die in car accidents than during childbirth) or fly on an airplane. As a living human being, you can't avoid risk.

And the risk in childbirth has been greatly overplayed. **Childbirth is not inherently risky,** even though the medical profession would like you to believe otherwise. This is how they make a living.

I will cover more specific concerns and solutions and preventions in another chapter later. For now, just know things can go wrong anywhere, at home or at the hospital. Sometimes there's something you can do about it, and sometimes there isn't. Knowing when you can help is the only step you can really take to prepare. But dwelling on possible misfortune won't make your pregnancy a happy one.

Having No Support

Sometimes we want to do something nobody else approves of. It could be a new hobby, a new career, moving to a new area, or giving birth unassisted. Whenever you do something new, there are usually others who've already done what you want to do. The tough part is you don't know any of those people yet, and your immediate family members and friends may think you're crazy.

Fortunately, how you give birth is your choice. You have to make all the decisions related to your pregnancy and your baby, since you're in charge. At least that's my hope for you. Ideally, your partner or another family friend is there to support you. But if all your immediate family members think a birth outside of the hospital—let alone an unassisted birth—is crazy, things may be a little more difficult for you.

Giving birth unassisted against the wishes of everyone you care about is difficult but possible. Many women who plan an unassisted birth don't tell everyone they know how they plan to give birth. More often than not, their partner is the only other person aware of their plans.

Depending on how strongly you feel about giving birth unassisted, you may have some other choices available to you. You could compromise and secure the services of a midwife. You can always choose not to call her when you're in labor.

Ideally, you'll discuss your birthing plans with your partner ahead of time. You never know how your partner will react until you broach the subject. Chances are he hasn't really thought much about it. You know him best, so you probably know how to approach him. You could slip tidbits of information into casual conversation, or you could tell him point blank you want to have this baby at home. You can stress the fact that childbirth is so natural women all over the world do it without help.

He may come around. It could take some time, so don't give up. It's in his best interest to have a healthy baby, and submitting yourself to hospital rules will not guarantee this for you. Don't expect your partner to shout with joy about your new birth plans. He's probably scared and wants to make sure you and the baby are healthy.

Giving birth is a major life event. While it's perfectly natural for your body to give birth, it's not something you do every day. Some women only do it once, and some women have lots of babies. But no matter how many babies you end up having, you will probably remember every birth. Therefore, your birth should happen the way you want it to. You'll only resent it later if you let your partner talk you into doing it in a different setting.

As long as you're prepared, you can deal with most problems that could arise (but most likely won't) just as well as a midwife could. If you need further assistance, you can go to the hospital. Besides, if something goes wrong, a midwife would transfer you to the hospital, too.

Technically, only the presence of two people is required at a birth: an expecting mother and her baby. However, sharing this intimate moment with your partner is wonderful. He can help you set up the room and clean up afterwards. But if you need to or want to, you're perfectly capable of doing it all by yourself. In fact, Laura Shanley gave birth to some of her children completely by herself. She preferred it that way.

By the way, if you need help during the birth, almost anyone can help you. In fact, most tasks can be accomplished by a child. And the things better left to an older child or adult, such as boiling scissors, are not time-sensitive.

Best of all, since there's no requirement to have an attendant at your birth at all, you get to choose who will be present. You may even decide you want someone to be available, but you'd prefer them to stay in the other room unless you call for assistance.

Do what feels right to you, but know you can always change your mind when you're in labor. I think it's a privilege to allow someone to witness the birth of your child. And you certainly don't need to allow anyone to stay just to please them. It's your birth, not theirs.

Legalities

Currently, there are several states in which a midwife-attended homebirth is illegal. Since laws change and there are a lot of states and countries, I encourage you to research the laws that apply to you.

However, even in areas which make it illegal to have a midwife-attended homebirth, **an unassisted birth is never illegal**.

As far as I can tell, Nebraska is the only state in the U.S. with a law slightly relevant to an unassisted birth. Apparently, it's a misdemeanor for the father to catch his own baby in a non-emergency situation.[29] However, the law doesn't forbid the mother or another family member to catch the baby. I'm not sure who came up with this law, but it seems pretty senseless. The important thing for you to know is even Nebraska law doesn't prevent you from having an unassisted birth at home.

Unassisted births are certainly discouraged in many "civilized" countries, but legal nonetheless. It would be hard to outlaw it, because sometimes women have unintentional unassisted births. For example, labor may progress too fast to get to the hospital or the midwife doesn't make it on time.

If you plan on having an unassisted birth, it may be advisable to keep those plans to yourself. Your family and friends may not be supportive. You can always tell them afterwards if you want to, or you can say "I didn't make it to the hospital in time". Alternatively, you can keep the entire birth experience to yourself if you feel more comfortable this way.

Getting legal documents for your newborn baby after having an unassisted birth may become a big hassle for you. But you have a right to get your baby's birth certificate and a social security card. Some states may require you to present proof of your pregnancy, or proof of a pediatric examination of the baby, or both. You may have to jump through a few other hoops as well. You can read more about getting a birth certificate for your baby in a later chapter. For now, just to know the paperwork hassle is not a reason to go to the hospital if you don't want to.

[1] Martin JA, Hamilton BE, Ventura SJ, et al. Births: Final data for 2010. National vital statistics reports; vol 61 no 1. Hyattsville, MD: National Center for Health Statistics. 2012.

2 Rebecca Flemming, Medicine and the Making of Roman Women (Oxford: Oxford University Press, 2000).

[3] Thomas, Laura (2011). "Empowered women shape modern maternity care" Retrieved from http://kaiserpermanentehistory.org/tag/prenatal-care/.

[4] Rooks, Judith (2006). "The History of Childbearing Choices in the United States" Retrieved from http://www.ourbodiesourselves.org/book/companion.asp?id=21&compID=75.

[5] Case, Christine L., Ed. D. (n.d.) "Handwashing" Retrieved from http://www.accessexcellence.org/AE/AEC/CC/hand_background.php.

[6] Wertz RW, Wertz DC. Lying-in: A history of childbirth in America. New York: Schocken Books. 1977

[7] Pregnancy and Childbirth around the World Blogspot. (2012) "Freebirthing, Dude!" Retrieved from http://pregnancyandchildbirtharoundtheworld.blogspot.de/2012/01/16-freebirthing-dude.html.

[8] New Zealand College of Midwives (2010) "The vaginal examination during labour: is it of benefit or harm?" Retrieved from http://www.thefreelibrary.com/The+vaginal+examination+during+labour%3A+is+it+of+benefit+or+harm%3F-a0251277462

[9] A randomized trial of increased intravenous hydration in labor when oral fluid is unrestricted. *Coco A, Derksen-Schrock A, Coco K, Raff T, Horst M, Hussar E.Fam Med. 2010 Jan; 42(1):52-6.*

[10] Romano, A. (2009). "First, Do No Harm: How Routine Interventions, Common Restrictions, and the Organization of Our Health-Care System Affect the Health of Mothers and Newborns". From the journal of perinatal education. Retrieved from http://www.ncbi.nlm.nih.gov/pmc/articles/PMC2730908/.

[11] Lamaze International (2008). "Avoiding Induced Labor Is More Beneficial To Moms And Babies." Retrieved from http://www.medicalnewstoday.com/releases/98156.php

[12] Natural Motherhood (2012). "Internal and External Fetal Monitoring Risks." Retrieved from http://www.natural-motherhood.com/external-fetal-monitoring.html.

[13] Smyth RMD, Markham C, Dowswell T. Amniotomy for shortening spontaneous labour. Cochrane Database of Systematic Reviews 2013, Issue 6. Art. No.: CD006167. DOI: 10.1002/14651858.CD006167.pub4

[14] Judy Slome Cohain. "Amniotomy and Cord Prolapse". Midwifery Today, Issue 108, Winter 2013.

[15] Henci Goer (2002). "Elective Induction of Labor". Revised and reprinted from Childbirth Instructor Magazine.

[16] Laura Kaplan Shanley: "Unassisted Childbirth"

[17] Lavender T and Mlay R. Position in the second stage of labour for women without epidural anaesthesia: RHL commentary (last revised: 15 December 2006). The WHO Reproductive Health Library; Geneva: World Health Organization.

[18] Henci Goer (1995). Ostetrics Myths Versus Research Realities: A Guide to the Medical Literature.

[19] American Journal of Epidemiology. (2001) 153 (2):103-107.doi: 10.1093/aje/153.2.103

[20] Downie, Andrew. (2001) "C-Sections in Vogue in Rio / Brazilian women see cesareans as faster and easier, but government tries to steer hospitals back to normal delivery". Retrieved from http://www.sfgate.com/health/article/C-Sections-in-Vogue-in-Rio-Brazilian-women-see-2956831.php.

[21] National Healthy Mothers (2012). "What You Need to Know About Cesarean Section: An Interview with Dr. Carol Sakala of Childbirth Connection." Retrieved from http://www.hmhb.org/virtual-library/interviews-with-experts/cesarean-section-c-section/.

[22] Martin JA, Hamilton BE, Ventura SJ, et al. Births: Final data for 2010. National vital statistics reports; vol 61 no 1. Hyattsville, MD: National Center for Health Statistics. 2012.

[23] Kim, Ben, Dr. (n.d.). "Vitamin K at Birth: To Inject or Not" Retrieved from http://drbenkim.com/vitamin-K-shot-baby.html.

[24] Bland (2009) Missouri Western State University. "The Effect of Birth Experience on Postpartum Depression". Retrieved from http://clearinghouse.missouriwestern.edu/manuscripts/59.php.

[25] Orgasmic Birth (n.d.). "What is Orgasmic Birth?" Retrieved from http://orgasmicbirth.com/about/what-is-orgasmic-birth/.

[26] Bastyr Center for Natural Health (2013). "Homeopathy Prevents Postpartum Hemorrhage". Retrieved from http://www.bastyrcenter.org/content/view/997/.

[27] Robin Elisse Weiss, LCCE (2014). "Postpartum Hemorrhage." Retrieved from http://pregnancy.about.com/cs/postpartumrecover/a/pph.htm.

[28] Margarett Scott, CPM. Three Keys to Avoiding Postpartum Hemorrhage. Midwifery Today Issue 48, Winter 1998.

[29] Shanley, Laura (2013). "Is Unassisted Childbirth Legal?" Retrieved from http://www.unassistedchildbirth.com/is-unassisted-childbirth-legal/.

Chapter 2

Your Pregnancy

How do you have a healthy pregnancy? Having a healthy baby inevitably requires you to be a healthy mother. We all know the basic don'ts: don't smoke, don't drink, and don't do drugs.

But is it enough to keep you and your baby healthy? Given there are plenty of sick people who don't smoke, drink, or do drugs, we can safely assume there's more to being healthy.

Health is a popular topic and widely written about. There's too much information about health rather than not enough. Here are the nutritional highlights for a healthy mother (and father):

- Eat a lot of (raw) fruits and vegetables
- Stay away from sugar, white flour, caffeine, and processed foods

A discussion on nutrition is beyond the scope of this book. And there are about as many opinions on what's healthy as there are people in this world. Some swear animal products make us unhealthy, especially products derived from unhealthy animals. Other sources cite the many problems with grains in our diet. Some even say too much fruit is unhealthy for you.

However, most people agree our bodies need a variety of vitamins and minerals to stay healthy. I encourage you to research what's good for you and your baby. You may even decide to consult with a nutritionist.

One way to decide what's healthy is to study the effects of certain diets on a group of people. Most people in the industrialized world don't eat a healthy diet. Therefore, as a population, we are sicker than others. Most populations who are robust and healthy don't eat processed foods. And when they eat meat or dairy products, they eat them fresh from healthy animals. Their diet also includes plenty of locally grown produce.

For your pregnancy and beyond, choose whole foods whenever you can. The best food is the type of food that doesn't come with a list of ingredients and is grown and harvested in an earth-friendly way.

As overwhelming as it seems, proper nutrition is only one aspect of health, albeit a big one. In addition to eating right, you need to exercise. If you haven't been active before, now is not the time to start a crazy workout routine.

At the very least, do some gentle stretches every day and go for a walk. When you stretch, stay off your back. Swimming is a great way to be active if you have the option. With any exercise, please don't overdo it. If you feel light-headed or out of breath, stop and rest. Drink plenty of water before, during, and after exercising.

Besides nutrition and exercise, other major areas affecting your health and overall well-being include:

- the presence of toxins in your life, such as in your food, your personal care products, and your home
- the time you spend outdoors (sunlight boosts your mood)
- the relationships you have with your friends and family (people are happier if they live in close-knit communities)
- having a great attitude

Prenatal Care

Why do we insist on prenatal care in the United States? First, let's talk about what prenatal care usually includes. In the first 28 weeks of pregnancy, prenatal visits take place every four weeks if you choose to see a medical provider. Between 28 and 36 weeks, you'll see your doctor or midwife every other week. Once you reach 36 weeks, appointments are scheduled weekly until you give birth. There may be additional visits, depending on your health and your provider's preferences.

Prenatal care includes many procedures, such as urinalysis, blood pressure check, tracking your weight, measuring your fundal height, blood tests, a vaginal swab, a glucose test, checking baby's heartbeat, and one or more ultrasounds. Some things are done at each appointment, for example, checking your blood pressure. Others only happen once, such as the vaginal swab. The goal of prenatal care is to ensure a healthy pregnancy and prevent or treat illnesses early.

You may have heard the following statement about prenatal care: people who don't receive prenatal care have a higher chance of preterm labor and low birth-weight babies. In reality, receiving prenatal care doesn't decrease your chances of preterm labor or low birth-weight babies at all.

Consider these findings by the Center of Disease Control on Prevention: The percentages of women who receive prenatal care goes down where the expecting mothers are unmarried, the pregnancy was unplanned, it's a teenage pregnancy, the women are not white, and/or they're part of a low socioeconomic group. Many women who don't receive prenatal care also don't have health insurance. Finally, some women wouldn't seek prenatal care, because they didn't want to draw attention to drug use or alcohol abuse[1].

These women are at risk for pregnancy complications *because of their circumstances*, not for lack of prenatal care. Teenagers and women of low socioeconomic groups are at a higher risk, with or without prenatal care. Teenage pregnancies carry a higher risk, because girls' bodies cannot handle pregnancies as well since they aren't fully developed yet. Similarly, women who are poor cannot afford to eat healthy. It's the circumstances which cause problems with their pregnancy and not that they didn't receive prenatal care. Those same circumstances might even prevent them from receiving prenatal care, for example, because they don't have health insurance.

As the same study showed, married women who planned to become pregnant are more likely to receive prenatal care. However, the reason their pregnancies turned out to be healthier is they were prepared to be pregnant, and therefore were more likely to take care of themselves.

The medical world certainly encourages you to seek prenatal care, but their reasoning behind it is flawed. And while obtaining prenatal care won't make you any healthier, it may give you a warm fuzzy feeling when, according to the doctor, everything is okay. Keep in mind, prenatal care will not prevent complications, just like merely going to the dentist regularly won't prevent cavities.

Are all the tests and check-ups during pregnancy truly necessary? If you've ever been to a prenatal appointment, it can certainly feel rather boring (unless it's an ultrasound where you get to see your baby). Does going to the doctor regularly really help you have a healthy pregnancy?

Since prenatal care mostly consists of checks and tests, it's important to know what the consequences of the tests results are. For example, if you had high blood pressure, your doctor might recommend a dietary change or medication to lower it. If your baby isn't growing according to schedule, there's probably not much your doctor can do about it.

When you decide if and how much prenatal care you want to receive, think about what the results would mean to you. You know how healthy you are, better than any doctor or midwife. You know what you need to do to be healthy. If you're not willing to change unhealthy habits, then all the medicine and check-ups in the world won't help you, either. You may even fall within the normal range regarding weight and blood pressure, but still not be in optimal shape for yourself.

Some things may be worth knowing, others may not be. If you wouldn't abort your pregnancy under any circumstances, then why should you even consider getting tested for possible infant deformities or disabilities? Those tests are not always accurate (they can give a false positive), and they create nothing but stress and worry.

According to John A. Haugen, "You do not need to do any screening or diagnostic testing. The benefits of any prenatal testing include reassurance, or in the event of a problem, preparation, optimal medical management, or termination of the pregnancy. The risks include additional worrying if you have abnormal screening tests but don't do diagnostic testing and the miscarriage risks associated with diagnostic testing. This risk of not doing any testing is not knowing about a birth defect, or a higher risk of one, before delivery."[2]

Finally, if you're the type who needs a lot of reassurance everything is going well, you can do most of the prenatal care on your own at home. You can always get a "second" opinion from a midwife or doctor if you're unsure or just need peace of mind.

Giving birth unassisted doesn't require you to go through pregnancy without regular prenatal care. You can choose to see a provider regularly throughout your pregnancy. But it's going to depend on your caregiver whether you tell them about your plans to give birth unassisted or not. Some caregivers may drop you as a patient for liability reasons.

Do-It-Yourself Prenatal Care

At the end of this chapter, I've included a sample schedule for DIY prenatal care. Change the weeks if you weigh yourself at week 11 of your pregnancy. You can either continue with week 14 or change it to 15. Starting at week 28, you can step on the scale every other week, then once a week after 36 weeks. You can weigh yourself less often if you prefer. The intervals I've chosen simply match most regular prenatal visits at a doctor's office.

The chart goes up to week 43, because pregnancies can last that long or even longer. Most likely, you'll have your baby before then. You may even be excited you're done "earlier" according to my chart. I didn't want to stop the chart at 40 weeks, because a lot of babies don't come on their due date (more on post-term pregnancies later).

Keeping Track of Weight Gain

Tracking weight gain is probably one of the easiest things you can do yourself during your pregnancy. Of course, you're going to gain weight (sorry to break it to you). But when you step on the scale, you need to keep all the variables the same. For example, you could always weigh yourself in the morning before you eat breakfast. While you can track your weight gain every week, you don't need to, especially during the first few months. Keep in mind, if you're suffering from morning sickness, you may lose weight in the first trimester.

How much weight should you gain? The amount of actual weight gain depends on several factors. The "normal" range is anywhere from 15 to 25 pounds. If you were underweight at the beginning of your pregnancy, you could stand to gain more weight. If you're overweight, you might gain less. Similarly, if you're carrying twins, you'll likely gain more. But as long as you gain weight slowly and steadily while eating a healthy diet, you'll be fine[3].

Keeping track of your weight on paper is not a bad idea, because it might help you keep yourself in check. At the end of your pregnancy, it can be tempting to sit on the couch and eat a lot of ice cream. This kind of indulgence, if it becomes a daily ritual, will lead to additional weight gain that most likely ends up on your hips.

Just so you know, pregnancy-related weight gain is distributed to your baby, the placenta, the amniotic fluid, your breasts, extra blood supply, stored fat for delivery and breastfeeding, and your enlarged uterus[4]. And because of this distribution, the amount of weight you gain won't be the best indicator of how much your baby is going to weigh at birth.

Checking Your Blood Pressure

We want your blood pressure to stay at a healthy level, because both low and high blood pressure can be a sign of trouble. According to the U.S. Department of Health & Human Services, your blood pressure should be 120/80. If your blood pressure is 140/90 or higher, then you have high blood pressure.[5]

Before you worry about the numbers, understand that blood pressure changes throughout the day. It's lowest when you're resting. Your blood pressure increases when you're nervous or agitated. That's why you may have higher blood pressure at a doctor's office than at home. Other things that affect your blood pressure, at least temporarily, include exercising, smoking, cold temperatures, caffeine, and certain medications.

To determine if your blood pressure is within normal limits, it needs to be measured at regular intervals over time. Since having high blood pressure can put you at risk for other problems, it's probably not a bad idea to monitor yourself periodically. Sometimes high blood pressure is the first sign something is wrong, but you can't tell if someone has it just by looking at them.

You can use an automatic or manual blood pressure cuff to check your own blood pressure at home. The manual version requires you to use a stethoscope, while the automatic version will display the numbers for you.

Your blood pressure is going to be a valuable indicator, especially towards the end of your pregnancy. Prevention is key. High blood pressure is usually caused by a combination of an unhealthy diet, insufficient exercise, and/or too much stress. Therefore, don't sit on the couch and eat chips all day, but don't work 60 hours a week or more, either.

For a more complete picture of your physical health, you can also measure your pulse. No equipment is necessary for this. Your pulse should be about 60 to 100 beats per minute. You can find your pulse on your neck or on the inside of your wrist. Once you find it, start the timer, and start counting. If you count for 30 seconds, multiply the result by 2 to get your pulse rate per minute. By the way, if you're an athlete, your heart might work more efficiently. If so, it may be normal for you to have a pulse rate lower than 60.[6]

Testing Your Urine

Medical providers will request a urine sample at every prenatal visit. Thankfully, it's easy to pee on demand when you're pregnant. But it might make you wonder why your urine should be tested so frequently.

The doctor is usually looking for glucose, protein, ketone, and bacteria. Finding high levels of one or more of those in your urine could be a sign something is wrong.

For example, high glucose levels could indicate gestational diabetes. The doctor will look for high levels or slightly elevated levels at more than one prenatal visit. High protein levels could show a urinary tract infection or preeclampsia (if accompanied by high blood pressure). If ketones are found, you may not be getting enough carbohydrates. Finally, bacteria can signal a urinary tract infection.[7]

You can easily test your urine at home. You can buy test strips and check your urine for these things and more, even including your PH levels. You can find test strips online, usually sold to diabetics.

Testing your urine is totally up to you. You may find it unnecessary, and it might be. A urinary tract infection rarely goes unnoticed. Your chances of gestational diabetes are a lot lower if you take care of yourself properly by eating a healthy diet. And if you can't keep food or liquids down, you probably know about it as well.

On the plus side, urine test strips are not expensive and the testing itself is not invasive at all. You may gain some peace of mind from them if you need it. Therefore, there's no reason not to test your urine at home, if you so desire.

Measuring Your Fundal Height

During pregnancy, a midwife or a doctor would keep track of the size of your uterus at each appointment. This is a more reliable way to find out how much your baby is growing than by tracking your weight gain. Fortunately, measuring your fundal height (the size of your uterus) is fairly easy to do on your own.

1. Empty your bladder
2. Lie on your back
3. Find your pubic bone right above your pubic hair
4. Feel for your uterus (at about 20 weeks, you'll find it at the level of your navel; later it will be higher up)
5. Measure the distance between the top of your pubic bone and the top of your uterus in centimeters (tape measures used for sewing are best for this purpose)

Measuring fundal height is not accurate until you're past 20 weeks of gestation. If you're about 20 weeks along, the top of your uterus will be at the level of your navel. As your pregnancy progresses, you'll find it above your navel.

The distance from the top of your uterus to your pubic bone should equal the gestational age of your baby. Therefore, if you're 26 weeks along, you would measure about 26 cm. If you're still having trouble doing this, I recommend looking at this article with illustrations online at www.wikihow.com/Measure-Fundal-Height.

Your measurement could be off by plus or minus 4 centimeters. If they're off by more, there are a couple of possibilities: you may have miscalculated your due date, or you may carry multiples. Keep in mind women often measure larger in second and subsequent pregnancies. Heavier women also tend to measure larger.[8]

Measuring your fundal height is a non-invasive procedure and a good indicator for fetal growth. It's most useful when it's done throughout your pregnancy. Obviously, you'll be looking for steady growth. At the end of your pregnancy, a decreased fundal height can tell you when your baby has dropped into the birth canal. And if you're concerned about your measurements, you can always make an appointment with a doctor or midwife.

Baby's Heart Rate

During your prenatal appointments, a midwife or doctor will listen to your baby's heartbeat. This is just another way of checking on your baby. You can do this yourself or with your partner at home, but it requires a little more skill than measuring your uterus.

Using a Stethoscope or Fetoscope

If you're using a stethoscope or fetoscope, you'll have to wait until you're further along in your pregnancy (20 weeks or later) to detect the baby's heartbeat. Start by lying down on your back and feel around for your baby's back. Your baby's spine is pretty long and hard and not too difficult to locate. Next, place the stethoscope in that area and listen.

It may be easier for your partner to find the heartbeat. However, it can take time and practice, even for a medically trained practitioner. A fetoscope uses the listener's forehead to conduct sound, meaning it's not a hands-off device and difficult to use continuously. It's partly why they're not widely used in the medical field.

To calculate your baby's heart rate, you need to time yourself as you count the beats. For example, you can count for 30 seconds and multiply the result by two. Your baby's heart rate should be between 120 and 160 beats per minute. If your count is below 100 beats per minute, you're most likely listening to your own heartbeat. Simply start over to find your baby's heart rate[9].

A stethoscope is fairly inexpensive, but it's difficult to use for a layperson. Additionally, it isn't really useful until about the time you feel your baby move, by which time you already know his heart is beating. Therefore, you may decide to skip monitoring your baby's heart rate altogether. In the end, it's totally up to you.

Using a Fetal Doppler

When you use a fetal Doppler, you can detect your baby's heartbeat a little earlier, because it uses ultrasound. To use the Doppler, start by spreading gel around your belly. Beginning about three inches below your navel, make small circles with your Doppler extending out until you find a heartbeat. The fetal Doppler will display the heart rate on its LCD screen[10]. Since the Doppler uses ultrasound, use it only sparingly, or preferably not at all (more on ultrasound and its risks soon).

Listening to your baby's heartbeat can be a fun bonding experience, especially for dads, since they don't get to feel the baby move. However, it's not absolutely necessary to check your baby's heart rate throughout your pregnancy. Even when you schedule regular prenatal care, your provider will only check your baby's heartbeat every four weeks until you get further along.

Blood Tests

Most of the blood tests performed during pregnancy check for various hormones and proteins in the mother's blood. The purpose of the tests is to find indicators for chromosomal abnormalities of the fetus.

If the tests results are positive, then further testing is required, for example, amniocentesis or chorionic villus sampling (CVS). Both tests are much more invasive and involve sampling amniotic fluid or placental tissue.[11]

If the initial blood test is negative, then your baby probably doesn't have Down syndrome or a neural tube defect. However, a positive or a negative result of the blood test is merely an indicator. Even amniocentesis and CVS are not 100% accurate in detecting problems with your baby. However, they do come with side effects and may even lead to a miscarriage.

According to a study by the World Health Organization, "the review shows that second-trimester amniocentesis significantly increased the risk of spontaneous miscarriage in women who underwent the procedure compared with those who did not." The study included 4606 Danish women with low risk of pregnancy loss.[12]

When testing for fetal abnormalities, there are only two options open to the expecting woman: either continue the pregnancy or abort it. If test results don't affect your chosen course of action, then you may not need to worry about getting tested.

When a woman continues a pregnancy where the baby probably has Down syndrome or another genetic disorder, she may choose to give birth in a hospital with a supportive NICU. The test results during pregnancy can give her time to prepare emotionally.

In conclusion, while getting your blood drawn is rarely harmful, it may not be necessary. I wouldn't recommend having it done for peace of mind, because the opposite may happen when you get a false positive. Otherwise, you don't have to consent to any blood draws if you don't want to.

Here are the most common things a provider would screen for during pregnancy:

- Blood type, Rh factor, and antibody screening
- Complete blood count
- Iron levels
- Rubella (German measles) immunity
- Hepatitis B testing
- Syphilis screening
- HIV testing
- Screening for down syndrome and other chromosomal abnormalities

Ultrasound

According to birth activist Beverly Beech, "The routine use of ultrasound in pregnancy is the biggest uncontrolled experiment in history." Chances are you've had at least one or more ultrasounds in your life. If you've been pregnant in the past, you most likely had at least one or possibly even several ultrasounds during each pregnancy.

OB/GYNs commonly use vaginal ultrasound at the first appointment to confirm the pregnancy. They check if the embryo is implanted in the uterus. They often do the next ultrasound at around 20 week's gestation. This time, ultrasound is used to determine the gestational age of the fetus and chart his or her growth. Many parents choose to find out the sex of the baby at this ultrasound. Another ultrasound is usually done if the woman's pregnancy continues past her due date to evaluate the amniotic fluid levels. Finally, if the medical provider suspects complications, they may order additional ultrasounds throughout the pregnancy.

What may surprise you is routine ultrasounds are not even recommended by any major organization. [13] Instead, ultrasound scanning is mainly a big business concern where marketing is important. Unfortunately, with the high prevalence of ultrasounds, many doctors have lost the ability to do things most midwives can do in their sleep. For example, doctors rely almost exclusively on ultrasound to ensure the proper growth of the fetus and to find out the position of the baby.

Many midwives who encourage natural childbirth use much simpler methods with the same precision. A midwife will measure the fundal height to check on your baby's growth, which you can do yourself by now. The practiced midwife can also feel for your baby and tell you where the head is located, without using ultrasound.

Most studies have shown ultrasound doesn't consistently reveal the fetal abnormalities it's supposed to detect. And a problem is often diagnosed in error. Even if a certain disease is diagnosed correctly in utero (of which we can never be 100% sure of), there's usually nothing that can be done for it, other than abort the pregnancy.

Another startling fact: "there are no federal radiation safety performance standards for diagnostic ultrasound." [14] There are no regulations on ultrasound machines or the technicians who use them, either. Each machine uses a different dose.

Here is what the FDA writes about ultrasound risks: "Even though there are no known risks of ultrasound imaging, it can produce effects on the body. When ultrasound enters the body, it heats the tissues slightly. In some cases, it can also produce small pockets of gas in body fluids or tissues (cavitation). The long-term effects of tissue heating and cavitation are not known." [15]

Today's equipment is even more powerful than the first-generation ultrasound machines. However, with the uncontrolled exposure from ultrasound, we have no idea what we're doing to our unborn children. According to Dr. Sarah Buckley's information, vaginal ultrasound is even more concerning in the first trimester. In her book, she states, "with vaginal ultrasound, there is little intervening tissue to shield the baby, who is at a vulnerable stage of development, and exposure levels will be high."[16]

You may believe ultrasound can diagnose problems ahead of time, and therefore, the use of ultrasound is justified. The most common reason for using ultrasound is to detect intrauterine growth retardation (IUGR) of the fetus.

But consider the following excerpt from Midwifery Today: "If doctors continue to try to detect IUGR with ultrasound, the result will be high false-positive rates. Studies show that even under ideal conditions, such as do not exist in most settings, it is likely that over half of the time a positive IUGR screening test using ultrasound is returned, the test is false, and the pregnancy is in fact normal. The implications of this are great for producing anxiety in the woman and the likelihood of further unnecessary interventions."[17]

Even if the prognosis for IUGR has become more accurate now than back in 1999, the screening still doesn't help. Intrauterine growth retardation cannot be prevented, changed, or stopped in most situations. The only exception would be a pregnant woman who is malnourished or using drugs.

To sum up, there seems to be no actual benefit to using ultrasound, because the diagnosis can miss defects or diagnose problems when there aren't any. Babies can be diagnosed much more accurately after birth, if there is a problem. And since most babies are healthy, it seems illogical to have every mother submit to routine ultrasound screening.

If the biggest problem with using ultrasound was the lack of obvious benefits, you would probably still use them, because most people currently believe they do no harm. However, "ultrasound adversely affects body tissues in three primary ways: heat, cavitation, and acoustic streaming."[18]

It may be difficult to know exactly how much harm they cause, partly because ultrasound machines and technicians differ widely. But why should we use ultrasound when we don't have to? Ultrasound scans may be the new x-rays, which were believed to be safe when they were first used on pregnant women.

Let's face it, the only reason most pregnant women gladly submit themselves to the ultrasound is they get to see their baby and find out the gender. You can measure growth just as accurately when you track your fundal height and your weight gain. Therefore, I invite you to put the mystery back into your pregnancy and find out your baby's gender when he or she is born.

All this being said, there's nothing wrong with scheduling an ultrasound if you so desire. Whether it's to reassure yourself you're not having twins (been there) or some other reason, you don't need to feel guilty about making this decision for yourself and your baby.

Pap Smears

Pap smears are done routinely once a year. During a pap smear, the doctor or midwife will take a sample of cells from your cervix or vagina. The primary reason for the Pap smear is to detect cancer. If your Pap smear results come back abnormal, the process might be repeated. The next step would be a biopsy.

A Pap smear is used to look for signs of infection or sexually transmitted diseases. However, a Pap smear is not a reliable indicator for sexually transmitted diseases. You need other tests to get conclusive results. But if you've been tested for STDs in the past, and you haven't been with any new partners since, there's probably no reason to get tested just because you're pregnant.

During prenatal care, another Pap smear is often done at the end of your pregnancy. This time, they take a sample from your vagina and your anus (but not from your cervix) to test for Group B Strep. Quite a few women are carriers of this type of bacteria without being ill. However, if the mother is positive, she can pass Group B Strep on to her baby. According to the Center of Disease Control and Prevention, a woman who tests positive but receives antibiotics during labor has 1 in 4,000 chance of having a Group B Strep positive baby. Without antibiotics, the odds are 1 in 200, which is still pretty low.[19]

You can purchase your own Group B Strep screening kit online, but you'll have to pay for the lab results. If you test positive, you then have a choice of antibiotics (usually administered via IV during labor) or alternative herbal remedies. Most homebirth midwives are familiar with this scenario. Therefore, testing positive for Group B Strep doesn't automatically require you to give birth in a hospital.

For your information, a baby affected by strep is going to display symptoms within days after birth. These symptoms can include lethargy, poor feeding, irritability, low or high heart rate, low blood pressure, low blood sugar, abnormal temperature, abnormal breathing, and lack of oxygen (blue or grey skin).[20] If you notice any of these symptoms in your baby, you need to take your baby to the hospital immediately.

There are plenty of women who decide the risks of antibiotics or herbal remedies outweigh the benefits. Other countries don't routinely administer antibiotics for Group B Strep, unless other risk factors are present, such as premature rupture of the membranes. There's only a slight chance of your baby getting sick, in which case you could treat him directly.

In conclusion, you can get tested for Group B Strep between week 35 and 37 of your pregnancy, if this really worries you. If the test results are positive, you can decide if you want to get antibiotics, try the herbal vaginal flush, or leave it alone. There will be more information about Group B Strep under the chapter "Pregnancy Concerns".

When it comes to Pap smears, many women who give birth unassisted skip this step. While the procedure itself doesn't seem to have any risks associated with it, having a doctor or midwife scrape samples from your cervix or vagina (depending on the test) can cause temporary bleeding and cramping. You also have to wait for test results, which means you won't actually know if you're Group B Strep positive on the day you give birth.

Putting It All Together

The Center for Unhindered Living has the following to say about prenatal care: "Then why do doctors insist you are putting your health and your baby's life at risk if you don't get prenatal care? First, if you decide not to get prenatal care, the doctor loses a lot of income. Second, if you realize that prenatal care is not necessary, it's not much of a stretch to decide that the presence of the doctor is not necessary at the birth either."[21]

Having an unassisted birth doesn't require you to do your own prenatal care. You have several options. First, you could find a midwife or doctor who will do your prenatal appointments. And while you may not find a doctor who is supportive of an unassisted birth, you could have better luck with a midwife.

Another option is to go to a doctor or midwife for all your prenatal appointments without letting them know you're planning an unassisted birth. You benefit by having a care provider you can call, even during labor if you want to. The drawbacks are you may have to pay for services you're not using. The most important thing about choosing a care provider is feeling comfortable with them. If you feel pressured into running tests you'd rather refuse, don't hesitate to switch providers.

It's up to you to decide what kind of testing you want to undergo and why. Some women trust the process and don't get tested at all. Others pick and choose which tests they want done. Women who have medical caregivers are more likely to get the entire battery of tests done than women who choose to give birth unassisted.

You could go through your entire pregnancy without checking much of anything. There's really no skill involved in growing a baby in your uterus. It happens on autopilot. Most likely, you'll check the scale out of curiosity, and as you get further along, you'll feel your baby move.

Finally, if you want to do your own prenatal care at home, you now have the knowledge to do so. You can follow the sample chart on the next page, or you can make your own. You can even create your own medical file and fill out a form during each of your check-ups, if you want to. It's up to you.

Weeks	Date	Weight	Blood Pressure	Fundal Height	Urine Results	Heart Rate (Baby)	Additional Testing
10				N/A			
14				N/A			
18				N/A			
22							Ultrasound
26							
30							Group B Strep
32							
34							
36							
38							
39							
40							
41							
42							
43							

Pregnancy Concerns

In this chapter, I will go over common pregnancy complaints. I'm probably not the first person to tell you that pregnancy comes with odd side effects, for lack of a better term. Even if you're healthy and doing everything right, pregnancy is going to bring about a few changes. Few women make it through with no complaints. Maybe we've earned the right to complain. Growing another human being is hard work.

Since you can have many of the problems at varying times throughout your pregnancy, this chapter is in purely alphabetical order. Here's the list of topics I'll be covering:

- Anemia
- Back pain
- Bathroom visits
- Cramps
- Diabetes
- Fatigue
- Getting sick
- Group Beta Strep
- Heartburn
- Hemorrhoids
- Hot flashes
- Hypertensive disorders
- Miscarriage
- Morning sickness
- Rhesus factor
- Shortness of breath
- Swelling (hands and feet)
- Thyroid disease

Anemia

Anemia is a common concern when you're expecting. During pregnancy, blood volume increases by 50%. To accomplish this, your body needs to produce more red blood cells. If there's not enough iron, you can quickly become anemic.

The symptoms of anemia include fatigue, shortness of breath, pallor, the desire to chew on nonfood items such as ice, a rapid heart rate, and ringing in your ears. There are two other types of anemia. Those are caused by a folate or Vitamin B^{12} deficiency[22]. Anemia is easily diagnosed with a simple blood test.

An anemic mother may have an increased risk for postpartum hemorrhage. Therefore, it's important to watch what you eat and increase your consumption of iron-rich foods. Fortified cereals are not the best choice because of their high sugar content. Instead, eat more red meat (preferably from grass-fed animals) and green, leafy vegetables.

Back Pain

During pregnancy and especially towards the end, you may experience lower back pain. You may also struggle with upper back pain. Both can be caused by the extra load you're carrying in the front. If you have back pain near your shoulder blades, you may be contributing to it with bad posture.

Unfortunately, there are no miracle cures for back pain, but there are many things you can do to prevent it and make it better. If you've been sedentary, start with some gentle stretches. Your stretches should be pregnancy-friendly, which means you need to stay off your back during your second and third trimester.

To make your back feel better, get moving every day. Even going for a walk can help. You don't have to run or walk fast to experience the benefits of exercise. In fact, be careful not to overexert yourself. Pay attention to your body's signals and take a break when you need one.

If your belly is not too big yet, you could try riding a stationary bike. However, I don't recommend riding an actual bike (unless you were an avid bike rider before your pregnancy), because you might tip over with your balance off-kilter. Swimming is another great way to get exercise. When you're in the water, there's no pressure on your back, and this feels great.

A heating pad can offer immediate pain relief or you can recruit your partner to give you a thorough back massage, possibly using topical pain relief. Another option is to schedule a prenatal massage with a massage therapist. If money is tight, ask someone else for the favor, maybe a close relative or a good friend.

As long as you stay active and stretch regularly, your back pain should be manageable. Of course, it's important to eat right to avoid gaining too much extra weight. Extra weight means any amount of weight you would have gained without being pregnant, for example, weight gain caused by eating three pizzas and two tubs of ice cream every evening.

Finally, make sure you're sleeping on a good mattress. Since we spend a lot of time asleep, you want adequate back support while you're in bed. If you wake up every morning with back pain, your mattress may be at fault.

The best sleeping position during pregnancy is to lie on your side with a pillow under your head and a pillow between your knees. You can use a small pillow underneath your growing belly for extra support. If you spend a lot of time sitting (for example at a computer), use good posture and consider investing in an ergonomic office setup.

Bathroom Visits

Going to the bathroom several times within one hour caused the most raised eyebrows from my older kids whenever I was pregnant. "You just went to the bathroom. Why do you have to go again?"

Increased bathroom visits can start in your first trimester. "Shortly after you become pregnant, hormonal changes cause blood to flow more quickly through your kidneys, filling your bladder more often. Also, over the course of your pregnancy the amount of blood in your body rises until you have almost 50 percent more than before you got pregnant. This leads to a lot of extra fluid getting processed through your kidneys and ending up in your bladder. Eventually, you may also feel pressure on your bladder from your growing uterus, which further compounds the problem."[23]

Besides avoiding diuretic beverages, there's nothing you can do about having to pee a lot. Fortunately, unless you're going camping, being close enough to a bathroom is not a difficult feat in the United States. Most stores have bathrooms, and you'll quickly find out which ones to frequent. You may even ponder the thought of publishing a book titled "The pregnant woman's favorite bathrooms in [insert your city]".

Please continue drinking plenty of water and going to the bathroom whenever you need to. Trying to hold it in can cause a urinary tract infection[24], while not drinking enough water will dehydrate you. And obviously, neither option is desirable or safe.

Colostrum

Colostrum is the milk your breasts produce for your newborn, but it can be present quite early. This is not a cause for concern. Some women report leaking colostrum in the fifth or sixth month. Every pregnancy is different, and you may never experience leaky breasts while you're pregnant. If you notice colostrum leaking, switch to nursing bras or use nursing pads in your regular bras to avoid getting wet spots on your shirts.

Cramps

In the first trimester, sometimes even before you know you're pregnant, you can experience cramps. Cramping refers to pain in your pelvic region which usually comes and goes. Many women deal with it every month during their period. Cramping can be anything from a minor annoyance to a downright painful experience.

In the first trimester, the embryo's implantation can cause cramps in your uterus. Your body is working hard to help your baby settle in. As long as cramps are not accompanied by bleeding, you can just let them run their course. A heating pad may help relieve the pain.

If cramps in the first trimester are accompanied by bleeding, you may have a higher risk of miscarriage. According to the American Pregnancy Association "Studies show that anywhere from 20-30% of women experience some degree of bleeding in early pregnancy. Approximately half of pregnant women who bleed do not have miscarriages."[25] [See section on miscarriage later]

Cramps may come to visit you again at the end of the third trimester. This is more likely with second and subsequent pregnancies, but it doesn't make them any more appealing. Although they may feel like cramps, we now call them Braxton Hicks contractions or false labor. You know this is not labor, because the contractions don't follow a pattern or increase in intensity. By the way, cramping at the end of your pregnancy is a sign your body is getting ready for labor, even though labor itself may still be a couple of weeks away.

Unfortunately, you'll have to put up with cramping after the pregnancy as well. These cramps are called afterpains. Afterpains stem from the uterus shrinking back to its original size. In the process, it does a little spring-cleaning.

Whenever you experience cramping, whether it's at the beginning or end of your pregnancy, do whatever it takes to make it more bearable. If you feel better walking around or changing positions, by all means do so. If resting makes you feel better, lie down and read a book or watch a movie. You could also take a warm bath or use a heating pad. For afterpains, many women find they need something stronger to help them cope, whether it's herbal remedies or over-the-counter Ibuprofen, but most of these are not safe to use during pregnancy.

Diabetes

A thorough discussion on diabetes type I and II is beyond the scope of this book. Type II diabetes usually requires lifestyle changes, while type I diabetes also requires the administration of insulin. Most midwives will not accept a patient with diabetes Type I.

If you were diagnosed with either type of diabetes, do your own research on how to treat and even reverse this disease. If your blood sugar is well under control, there may be little reason to give birth at the hospital. Whether you feel comfortable giving birth unassisted at home is totally up to you.

Some women are diagnosed with gestational diabetes during their pregnancy. According to the Mayo Clinic, the potential risks associated with gestational diabetes include a large baby, a preterm baby, and a baby with low blood sugar. Your child may also be more likely to develop Type II diabetes later in life. Gestational diabetes increases your own risk of high blood pressure and preeclampsia and future diabetes.[26]

Medical providers administer a glucose tolerance test to every pregnant woman during the second trimester to rule out gestational diabetes. Positive test results may lead to additional monitoring of mother and baby and possibly an early induction of labor.

You can purchase an in-home glucose tolerance test online if you desire. I encourage you to read the label of ingredients before you drown that beverage. It may not be something you want to put into your body. Alternatively, you can buy the prick-your-finger glucose monitors, which are relatively inexpensive. You can check your blood sugar first thing in the morning and even a few times throughout the day to make sure you're in the normal range.

With diabetes, gestational or otherwise, there are a lot of things you can do to heal your body naturally, mostly through diet and lifestyle. And while I have found no official studies on naturally curing Type I diabetes, there are accounts of people who have done it on their own, which leads me to believe it's possible.

If you have gestational diabetes, it's a good idea to work with a nutritionist. The key to keeping your blood sugar stable is to eat small meals frequently throughout the day and to include the right ratio of protein and carbs.

Fatigue

You can feel fatigued anytime during your pregnancy, but most women feel noticeably more tired during the first and last trimester. During the first three months, your body is essentially building most of your baby's body parts. Your body is doing some rearranging to make room for your growing uterus. You've also taken on the new task of nourishing your baby and managing her waste products. This is strenuous, even though not visibly so. When you feel worn out, take the hint and rest whenever you can. Go to bed early or take naps during the day.

In your second trimester, you'll probably have fresh bursts of energy, and many women feel wonderful during this time. Morning sickness is usually over and your body has adjusted to its new job. However, during the third trimester, the fatigue comes back with a vengeance as the weight of the baby is really putting some pressure on your body.

As difficult as it can be for many women, it's a good idea to put your feet up as much as possible. You need to let go of trying to accomplish everything. Once your baby is there, that's a thing of the past, anyway. Your partner knows how to use the dishwasher and the washing machine. Just let him go without clean underwear, and he'll figure it out.

Getting more sleep than your usual eight hours is important during pregnancy. Going to bed early may seem like you're wasting time, but you'll feel so much better if you get enough rest. Your sleep will probably be interrupted, because it's difficult to get comfortable with a watermelon-belly and constant trips to the bathroom.

Don't do everything you normally do by increasing your caffeine consumption. It's much better and healthier to get extra rest for both you and your baby. Avoid sugar highs as well, because they don't help you get the rest you need, either.

Getting Sick

Being sick stinks, whether you're pregnant or not. However, when you're expecting, you need to stay away from certain medications, prescription, and over-the-counter medicine. You definitely won't be able to take Ibuprofen, Aspirin, or Pepto-Bismol while you're pregnant. You may not even be able to take cough medicine and a variety of other products.

Most pharmaceuticals include a warning for pregnant and nursing women. If you're not sure, ask a doctor or a pharmacist. Remember, some herbal remedies and essential oils can be even more potent than prescription drugs. Therefore, please proceed with care. Both prescription drugs and alternative medicine can be dangerous, especially if they're not used correctly.

If you feel a cold coming on, you might try taking extra Vitamin C or eating foods with a high Vitamin C content. For a headache, a cold washcloth on your forehead, a darkened room, and/or eating an apple can bring relief. Similarly, you can ease other pain or discomfort without ingesting drugs of any kind.

Group Beta Strep

You've probably heard of Group Beta Strep, short GBS. Most women have these bacteria present in their vagina. Pregnant women are usually tested for GBS close to the end of their pregnancy, between 36 and 37 weeks.

The interesting thing about GBS is that the test results vary from day to day. You may test positive for GBS one day and negative the next. But because you have to wait for results, this test has to be done well before you go into labor. And even though most women have some GBS bacteria present, most babies don't get sick.

If these other risk factors are present, it may be more likely for your baby to get sick:

- Your baby is born before 32 weeks
- Your water was broken for more than 18 hours
- You developed a fever during labor
- You had a urinary tract infection during your pregnancy[27]

The prescribed treatment for any women who tests positive with GBS is the administration of antibiotics through an IV during labor. Naturally, there's no guarantee the antibiotic will work. Babies can still get sick even if you receive this treatment.

Many people dislike antibiotics for various reasons, but there's an alternative treatment available. It's called chlorhexidine (Hibiclens) and used as a douche during labor. As a preventive measure, you can take probiotics and consume raw garlic with your meals. This will reduce the buildup of these bacteria.

Most infections caused by GBS occur within the first week of life. Signs of such an infection in your newborn baby may include:

- Difficulty breathing
- Fever
- Jaundice
- Poor feeding
- Vomiting

- Seizures
- Swelling of the abdomen
- Bloody stools[28]

If you notice any of these signs in your newborn, seek medical attention for her right away, whether it's caused by a GBS infection or something else.

Since neither the test results nor the prescribed treatment can guarantee a healthy baby, some women decide to forgo testing altogether.

Just so you know, according to the Centers for Disease Control and Prevention, in 2012 the average number of newborns with early onset (occurring during the first week of life) Group B Strep was 0.25 per 1,000.[29] That's one baby in 4,000 births. The vast majority of these babies can be treated successfully. However, this study didn't differentiate between mothers who had been treated for GBS and those who hadn't.

The odds are on your side, whichever way you decide to handle this. You can get tested for GBS at a doctor's office. You can even perform this test yourself and send it off for results. Keep in mind, it takes a few weeks to get the results, so this needs to be done well before your due date.

Heartburn

Heartburn, a burning sensation traveling up your esophagus and throat, is somewhat like drinking a caffeinated beverage and then burping, but a lot less pleasant. It can actually be very uncomfortable and even painful. Heartburn can come anytime, day or night. As your stomach is pushed up higher by your growing uterus, heartburn may become more of a problem as pregnancy progresses.

There are a few strategies which can help relieve heartburn. Eating small meals is one of them. You may also want to avoid fried, spicy, or rich foods. Avoiding drinking a lot during meals and don't lie down directly after eating. Use trial-and-error to find out which foods trigger heartburn for you. Then you can aim to avoid those foods or eat less of them.

Heartburn can be worse at night when you're lying down. Sitting up seems to relieve it. This is why many elderly people like to sit in those big armchairs, and some people even sleep in them. There are some over-the-counter meds you can take to relieve heartburn, but I don't know if they would really do you any good. Supposedly, they don't do any harm. However, you need to verify they're safe to take if you absolutely want to try medication for this annoying side effect of pregnancy.

Relief from heartburn will come at the end of your pregnancy, and possibly even before you give birth. You may experience lightening, which means your baby has descended into the birth canal, a few days or weeks before labor begins. While the baby's new position will put more pressure on your bladder, increasing the frequency of bathroom visits, it should relieve your stomach and lungs. You may feel less out of breath, and you may not experience heartburn anymore, or at least less often and less severely.

Hemorrhoids

Hemorrhoids are located in your anal canal. They can become swollen or inflamed, causing itching, pain, or bleeding. This sounds worse than it is. Having hemorrhoids feels like having little bumps around your anus, which are sensitive to the touch.

Hemorrhoids can be healed by keeping your stools soft. If you're suffering from constipation, drink more water, increase your fiber intake, and get physically active. Avoid straining on the toilet because that makes hemorrhoids worse. And while poor lifestyle choices can encourage hemorrhoids, they're more prevalent during pregnancy because of the extra weight pushing down on your anal canal.

The good news is hemorrhoids can be avoided or at least reduced by taking above measures. You won't automatically get hemorrhoids just because you're pregnant. But if you get them, rest assured you're not alone.

Besides keeping your stools soft, you can try a sitz bath. You don't have to purchase anything special to do this. The word 'sitz' comes from the German word 'sitzen' and just means 'to sit'. Simply fill your tub with warm water and sit in it for 20 to 30 minutes. Afterwards, it should feel a little better, and you can repeat a sitz bath as often as you like.

Hemorrhoids can appear several months before your baby is born. Unfortunately, they don't disappear immediately at birth. Instead, they stick around for a few more weeks. Even though hemorrhoids are quick to appear and slow to go, you should consult a doctor if the pain or bleeding is severe, if you're soiling yourself with stool, or if your hemorrhoids don't get any better down the road[30].

Hot Flashes

Many women experience hot flashes throughout their pregnancy. Hormonal changes and the increased blood supply are at fault. You're more likely to sweat during the second and third trimester. Unfortunately, it doesn't end there. Most likely, you'll still be sweating postpartum, because your body has to get rid of the extra fluids.

In addition to hormonal changes, you're carrying around extra weight in the front, which will end up being about the size of a watermelon. It's a pretty good workout.

There's not a lot you can do about feeling hot except for dressing in layers, allowing you to shed some clothes if you need to cool down. Stay hydrated. Finally, take pity on your partner. If he has blue lips, have mercy and ease up on the air conditioning. You can also use fans at your desk and by your bed to keep cool. Finally, you could take a cold shower in the middle of the day or, if you have the option, you can go swimming.

Hypertensive Disorders

Preeclampsia can be a pretty serious pregnancy condition. A woman with preeclampsia has high blood pressure, protein in her urine, and swollen hands and feet. Therefore, both blood pressure and urine are checked regularly throughout your pregnancy.

A woman with preeclampsia may develop eclampsia. This is a condition in which the woman will have seizures. Unfortunately, the best way to get rid of preeclampsia is to give birth. But since women can get preeclampsia starting at week 20 of their pregnancy, inducing labor is usually not the best choice until you're much closer to your due date.

A doctor may recommend bed rest for a woman with preeclampsia. Other treatment options may include giving baby aspirin or calcium. The problem with preeclampsia is that blood flow to the placenta is compromised, which puts your baby at risk.

Your risk for preeclampsia goes up if you're overweight, under 20 or over 40 years of age, are carrying multiples, or have diabetes or other medical conditions[31]. While you can't influence your age or the number of babies you're carrying, you can certainly be proactive about your health.

Preeclampsia may be prevented and avoided almost entirely by exercising regularly and eating an exceptionally good diet. High blood pressure is often the first indicator of preeclampsia, but it's not the only one. One high blood pressure reading isn't necessarily a cause for concern. But according to the Mayo Clinic, "Blood pressure that is 140/90 millimeters of mercury (mm Hg) or greater — documented on two occasions, at least four hours apart — is abnormal."[32]

Can you still give birth unassisted if you have high blood pressure? It depends entirely on what you feel comfortable with and whether you have any other symptoms. If high blood pressure is accompanied by sudden swelling, severe headaches, loss of vision, abdominal pain, nausea, vomiting, decreased urination, protein in your urine, or shortness of breath[33], seek immediate medical care.

Miscarriage

Miscarriages are a lot more common than you might think. While certain factors may contribute to a woman's miscarrying, each pregnancy is unique. Most of the time, doctors and midwives cannot explain why a particular miscarriage took place.

During a miscarriage, the process of building a little human is disrupted and can't be completed correctly. Therefore, your body aborts the pregnancy. When your fetus dies and pregnancy ends before 20 weeks, it's called a miscarriage. If the baby dies in utero after 20 weeks, it's called a stillbirth.

During a miscarriage, depending on when it happens, you'll have cramps and vaginal bleeding. When you miscarry before 12 weeks (which is when most miscarriages occur), you will pass a lot of blood clots, followed by more bleeding, similar to a strong period. Depending on the length of gestation, you may not even be able to distinguish the fetus.

If a doctor determines your baby is not alive (for example, during a prenatal ultrasound), he may offer you medication to induce your body to abort the pregnancy sooner. As with inducing a full-term pregnancy, there shouldn't be any need to do so. If the fetus is not alive, your body will expel it on its own. However, this can take time, which is why women often elect to induce as opposed to continuing the pregnancy with a dead fetus. The induction may help bring closure and reduce trauma.

However, one reason not to agree to a D&C (dilation and curettage—the procedure of removing tissue from inside your uterus) is your baby might be just fine. Ultrasound is notoriously unreliable, as I have explored in an earlier chapter. Therefore, it's possible for a doctor to misdiagnose a miscarriage, when in fact the baby is perfectly healthy.

It happens more often than you'd think.[34] There are women who decided to miscarry naturally at home after a devastating ultrasound diagnosis, but instead continued their pregnancy with no problems and gave birth to a healthy baby several months later. The bottom line is when you choose a D&C, you risk terminating a potentially viable pregnancy.

There are other reasons to refrain from a vaginal ultrasound. Ultrasound raises many concerns and potentially causing a miscarriage is just one of them. This is what Beverly Beech has to say about ultrasound and miscarriage: "It is ironic that women who have had previous miscarriages often have additional ultrasound examinations in order to 'reassure' them that their baby is developing properly. Few are told of the risks of miscarriage or premature labour or birth."[35]

While the cramping can be painful, it's easier to bear the physical anguish of a miscarriage than the emotional one. It's a devastating loss, and you may go through all the stages of grief for quite some time. Your body knows what to do during a miscarriage and afterwards, but you have to give your heart time to heal. It's up to you to decide if and when you want to try to have another baby.

Some women have several miscarriages in a row and still go on to having a healthy baby afterwards. Others stop trying. There's nothing wrong with either choice. Give yourself time to heal and grieve. The grieving process can be short or long, because everyone is different.

Morning Sickness

Many women experience morning sickness, especially during the first trimester. Some women have a hard time keeping food down for the entire duration of their pregnancy, and they end up losing weight. While there are quite a few recommendations on how to cope with morning sickness, there's no miracle cure.

You can try eating salty foods, such as crackers. While they have very little nutritional value, this kind of food often seems to help with nausea. It also helps to eat small meals. Finally, you can use the trial-and-error method to find out which foods offend you, and hopefully, there are a couple left that don't.

For most women, morning sickness disappears or at least lessens during the second trimester. In the meantime, take it easy. Don't expect to accomplish the things you used to do before you got pregnant. If you spend half your day in the bathroom, you won't have the energy to do much else.

If you experience severe nausea and can't even keep liquids down, you may need medical assistance. Signs of dehydration include dark urine (or no urine at all), headaches, dizziness, fatigue, and chapped lips. If you think you might be dehydrated, please go to the doctor.

Rhesus Factor

About 15% of the population is Rh negative.[36] Normally, this isn't a concern. However, during pregnancy, it can become an issue. The blood stream of the mother can mix with that of the baby. Since they're potentially not compatible when the mother is Rh negative, this can have several consequences, for example, miscarriage, abortion, or an ectopic pregnancy. Finally, if there's a fall or an accident, it can lead to placental abruption or uterine bleeding.

I know this sounds terrifying. Fortunately, it's easy to find out if you're Rh negative (a simple blood test) and seek treatment. An Rh-positive mother can receive RhoGAM (Rh immune-globulin).

RhoGAM prevents the creation of antibodies against the baby's positive Rh factor. If there's no treatment before the birth, your baby may have jaundice, lethargy, or low muscle tone. Breastfeeding and bilirubin lights can help. Unfortunately, in more severe cases, there may be brain damage or even death of the infant.

The biggest problems occur during subsequent pregnancies. If the Rh-negative mother becomes sensitized, a new Rh-positive baby would be at great risk, because of the antibodies already present in the mother's blood.

Fortunately, chances of the bloodstreams mixing are slim, outside of a traumatic event. But definitely find out whether you're Rh negative, just in case. Afterwards, you need to decide what you want to do about it. But even if you need RhoGAM, you might still give birth at home with the help of a supportive midwife.

According to the American College of Obstetricians and Gynecologists, Rh immunoglobulin has to be given to the woman before she becomes sensitized. This means, it needs to be done within 72 hours after giving birth to an Rh-positive child.[37] While not doing this may not affect the child you're currently carrying, it can become a problem for future children who are Rh positive.

While RhoGAM shots are now being administered during pregnancy in the United States at 28 and 36 weeks, there are quite a few safety concerns about them. First, RhoGAM shots often contain mercury. There is a mercury-free version available and has been since 1996, but you may not get the mercury-free version from your doctor. Second, RhoGAM is a blood product. However much it's cleaned up, there are still risks associated with injecting other people's blood into your body.

If you're going to opt for a RhoGAM shot, it makes sense to wait until after the birth. If your baby is also Rh negative, then you don't need to get a shot. The baby's blood type can be determined by sampling the cord blood. You can even do this at home if you procure a test kit beforehand.

If both parents are Rh negative, there's no need to worry about this topic. Here, the baby will also be Rh negative and therefore compatible with your blood type. RhoGAM will be completely unnecessary.

Just so you know, it's highly unlikely for the mother's and baby's bloodstream to cross paths. In utero, the blood streams don't normally mix. And during a gentle birth without interventions, this isn't likely to happen, either. The risk goes up if you're undergoing:

- An induced abortion or menstrual abstraction
- An ectopic pregnancy
- Chorionic villus sampling
- Amniocentesis
- A blood transfusion

If you are Rh negative, you have to decide. RhoGAM shot: yes or no. If yes, will you have it done during pregnancy or wait until after birth? The least invasive option is to get the shot after the birth if your baby is Rh positive. However, some women decide against RhoGAM. If this is your choice, make sure nobody pulls on the cord and allow the placenta to arrive on its own time.

Rh-negative women who are expecting a subsequent child after having given birth to an Rh-positive child may have become sensitized. If this applies to you, you can get tested for antibodies to help you make a decision and determine the best care for yourself and your new baby.

There are risks associated with doing nothing and with getting the RhoGAM shot. Further discussion on the topic is necessary to understand the pros and cons of each option. I absolutely encourage you to do additional research. For starters, I recommend reading "Anti-D in Midwifery: Panacea or Paradox?" by Sara Wickham.

Shortness of Breath

You may not be able to keep up with your kids or even do small household chores, especially at the end of your pregnancy. All the tasks you normally took care of quickly and easily will seem more cumbersome. As your uterus is expanding to make room for your growing baby, your stomach and your lungs are getting squished. Naturally, this will cause you to feel short of breath.

Take frequent breaks and delegate some of your chores to your other kids, and don't forget to involve your partner. Someone else can vacuum for a while.

When I was pregnant, my kids really enjoyed helping me. For example, they loved closing my sandals for me, because feet are so hard to reach at the end of pregnancy. If I dropped something, I would usually ask them to pick it up for me. Now they're used to the idea that everyone—even mommies—need help sometimes.

You probably don't want to start any new strenuous activities, such as mountain climbing or playing tennis. Depending on your pre-pregnancy fitness level, you can probably continue doing what you used to do, but don't expect to keep up the same intensity until the very end.

If you were very active before you got pregnant, you may not feel short of breath. If you're carrying low, you may not feel short of breath, either. Instead, you may spend more time in the bathroom. Deep breathing is also easier once your baby drops, which may happen before you go into labor. If nothing else, you get to take some deep breaths again once your baby is born.

Finally, shortness of breath can be attributed to other causes, such as anemia.[38] If you suspect this, some simple blood work can put your mind at ease, allowing you to supplement as needed.

Swelling (Hands and Feet)

Even though the uterus is nowhere near your feet and hands, both can become swollen when you're carrying a baby. During pregnancy, your body produces more fluids than ever, and for various reasons: fluid retention, weight gain, and the hormone relaxin. The fluid and extra water retention make your feet, hands, and ankles swollen.

The swelling should disappear within a few days of giving birth. Until then, you probably won't be able to wear a ring, and you may have to steal your partner's shoes. It's even possible for your shoe size to increase permanently.

In the summer, the heat can make swelling worse. Stay hydrated and cool down whenever you get the chance. It's possible for your hands or feet to swell up temporarily if you get too hot outside. The swelling should subside fairly quickly once you get to a cooler area.

While your hands and feet may feel more swollen at different times of the day, they tend to swell up gradually. If you experience any sudden or excess swelling or swelling in your face or around your eyes, especially at the end of pregnancy, see a healthcare professional as soon as possible. This could be a sign of preeclampsia, which is very serious.

Thyroid Disease

Even if you've been diagnosed with hypothyroidism or hyperthyroidism, you can still have an unassisted birth. However, you need to see a doctor regularly to ensure your dosage is correct. During pregnancy, your hormone levels change a lot, which affects your thyroid hormones as well. As long as you follow your doctor's instructions and get your dosage adjusted, you shouldn't have any problems.

As soon as you find out you're pregnant, schedule an appointment and get your blood drawn. Your dosage will probably be adjusted. Your practitioner will recommend another blood draw during your second trimester. Afterwards, your thyroid hormones should remain fairly stable throughout the rest of your pregnancy.

By about six weeks postpartum, your thyroid hormone levels will have returned to your usual pre-pregnancy levels. Schedule another blood draw and get your dosage adjusted accordingly.[39] An under- or overactive thyroid will merely result in additional blood draws and a change of your daily hormone dosage. However, you can't skip those extra check-ups, because they're extremely important for you and your baby. By the way, midwives usually can't prescribe medications. There's still no need to go to an OB/GYN for this, just because you're pregnant. Your primary doctor can continue to prescribe your thyroid hormones for you.

High-Risk Pregnancy

Some women plan a midwife-attended homebirth but over the course of their pregnancy, the midwife determines it's too risky. The reasons for this vary. You may have been diagnosed with gestational diabetes or high blood pressure, or you may have exceeded your due date by too many days.

Midwives usually have to meet certain guidelines to keep their license to practice. In short, there's no use arguing with them even if you feel perfectly safe continuing with your homebirth plans. If your midwife drops you from her care, you basically have two options available to you: you can give birth at a hospital or you can give birth at home on your own.

If your midwife already works with a doctor who understands your wishes for a natural childbirth, then you're probably in excellent hands at the hospital. In case of a transfer, your midwife may still come with you to support you, even though she won't be in charge of your care.

If your midwife doesn't work with a doctor, you may end up seeing whoever is available. The outcome depends on the type of doctor and their views on natural childbirth. Some hospital staff are very understanding when a woman planning a homebirth ends up under their care. They try to help her give birth as naturally as possible. Unfortunately, some medical professionals can be hostile towards a mother who planned a homebirth.

It helps to ask around in your area. Which hospital is the friendliest toward natural childbirth? Which doctor is the most supportive? Find out early during your pregnancy, just in case.

The other option I mentioned is giving birth at home without a care provider. I have done just that myself. Now I don't recommend doing this if you're considered high risk. However, I know medical professionals don't always think alike, and it's deceptively easy to be labeled as high risk when you really aren't.

For example, during my second pregnancy, I had an OB/GYN who considered me to be high risk. He based it on the fact I had given birth prematurely with my first child (36 weeks and 4 days) and that she was small (4 pounds even). As a result, during my second pregnancy, this doctor scheduled numerous ultrasounds to assess the baby's growth.

When I switched to a midwife, she didn't think I was high risk. And the baby was born after 41 weeks and 3 days, weighing a healthy 8 lbs. 4 oz. All my unassisted births were post-term pregnancies (43+2, 43+6, 42+5), and no midwife would have attended my births, merely because they were late.

It can be even more difficult to find a supportive care provider if you exhibit some risk factors in combination. For example, if you've had a C-section and display signs of high blood pressure or high blood sugar, then you're considered even riskier than a woman who had a previous vaginal birth and high blood pressure or high blood sugar.

Still, you decide how you give birth. But you shouldn't make this decision lightly. Educate yourself about your options, so you can make the choice that's right for you and your baby.

How to Have a Natural Birth at the Hospital

There's a possibility your midwife cannot be your provider at your birth, and you end up giving birth at a hospital. Sometimes, women transfer to the hospital, even though they had planned to give birth unassisted at home. There can be several reasons for this decision. Here is the good news: a natural birth is entirely possible at the hospital.

It might be devastating to have your birth plans derailed, but the hospital can be a safer option for some women. And even though you may give birth at the hospital, you probably still want to have your baby as naturally as possible. To do this, you need a plan.

1. Know What You Want

It's not enough to want to give birth naturally. You must understand why you want things to be a certain way. Know the most common interventions and decide which ones are worth fighting against. For example, you may not want to have any IV fluids, but you could compromise by having the IV ready to go just in case.

2. Write It Down

Lots of women write up a birth plan to ensure they're getting the birth they envision. Ideally, the hospital staff takes the time to read your birth plan and help you do things your way, but that's not realistic. If anyone reads your birth plan, they'll probably just skim it. Your best bet is to keep it short, sweet, and to the point.

You can write down what you don't want in bullet form, or you can write what you want for your birth. Having it in writing will also help your support person make your case for you when you can't talk for yourself. And it will remind you why you really don't want to have an epidural etc.

3. You Need a Support Person

You may be strong and confident and great about standing up for yourself most of the time. But when you're in labor, you're vulnerable. You may be scared, nervous, worried, or just distracted by the beautiful process of labor and childbirth. That's why you need someone with you at the hospital who will stand up for what you want. It could be your partner, your midwife, a doula, or your mother. Ideally, find someone who is diplomatic enough they won't antagonize the hospital staff but also someone who's got your back.

4. Avoid Being Antagonistic

As much as I don't like hospitals, I know being antagonistic won't help you get the type of care you desire. It's much better to be nice and kind about your requests. If your requests are being ignored, then you may have to be more assertive, but it's always better to ask nicely first.

And sometimes, it's better to ask for forgiveness later than to get permission. For example, if you're hungry or thirsty and the hospital doesn't allow you to eat or drink, have your support person sneak food in. The nurses won't bend the rules for you however nicely you ask them to. The same is true for walking around during labor. If you're not hooked up to anything, just move about as much as you want.

5. Go in at the Right Time

If your water has broken but labor hasn't started yet, wait to go to the hospital unless you're running a fever. After your water has broken, the hospital puts you on the clock. Most likely, you'll have to give birth within 12 or 24 hours. Otherwise, they'll perform a C-section. Even if you show up in labor at a later time, it may not be a good idea to tell them your water has been broken for more than a day.

Similarly, if you're overdue, wait for labor to start, unless there are other complications. Your baby will come when he's ready.

If you plan on having a vaginal birth after Caesarean (VBAC) even though the hospital isn't supportive of VBACs, show up at the hospital ready to push. The same is true if you're having a breech baby.

Coming in too early often results in additional unnecessary interventions. Hospital staff is unlikely to send you home if your water has broken or your due date has passed. That means they'll induce labor. But you already know when inducing labor doesn't work, you may end up with a C-section.

If you live far away from the hospital and worry about giving birth in the car by waiting to go in, hang out in the parking lot of the hospital during labor. Alternatively, you could go for a walk around the neighborhood with your partner or go to another place nearby. This way, you're close for when you need medical attention, but the clock hasn't officially started ticking yet.

6. Trust Your Instincts

It's difficult to tune out when you're in a busy, brightly lit room. But even though the hospital staff is close by and telling you what to do, it's important to trust your instincts. Your body knows how to give birth, even if you've never done it. If you feel like walking around, you need to do so. If you feel like resting, lie down. If you're hungry or thirsty, eat and drink. I know hospitals often have rules forbidding all these things, but those rules make little sense. They certainly won't help you give birth naturally the way you want to.

7. *Ask Someone to Watch Your Baby*

Once your baby is born, the hospital staff will focus on administering various treatments to your newborn. If you're attached to a fetal monitor or an IV or being treated for vaginal tears, you can't watch over your baby. Have your support person stay with him to make your wishes known and ensure they're being complied with. And as soon as possible, demand to hold your baby. You and your baby need to get to know each other.

In conclusion, the more you know about childbirth and what you truly want, the easier it will be to have a natural birth at the hospital. You can totally do this!

---

[1] Kiely & Kogan, (n. d.) "Reproductive Health of Women – Prenatal Care." Retrieved from
http://www.cdc.gov/reproductivehealth/ProductsPubs/DatatoAction/pdf/rhow8.pdf

[2] Haugen, John A. (n.a.) "The Facts on Prenatal Testing." Retrieved from http://www.haugenobgyn.com/prenatal_testing.aspx?AspxAutoDetectCookieSupport=1.

[3] WebMD (2013). "Gain Weight Safely During Your Pregnancy." Retrieved from http://www.webmd.com/baby/guide/healthy-weight-gain.

[4] WebMD (2013). "Gain Weight Safely During Your Pregnancy." Retrieved from http://www.webmd.com/baby/guide/healthy-weight-gain.

[5] Agency for Healthcare Research and Quality (2012). "Measuring Your Blood Pressure at Home: A Review of the Research for Adults." Retrieved from http://effectivehealthcare.ahrq.gov/index.cfm/search-for-guides-reviews-and-reports/?productid=894&pageaction=displayproduct.

[6] Laskowski, M.D. (2013) "What's a normal resting heart rate?" Retrieved from http://www.mayoclinic.com/health/heart-rate/AN01906.

[7] The American College of Obstetricians and Gynecologists (2014). "FAQ – Routine Tests in Pregnancy". Retrieved from http://www.acog.org/-/media/For-Patients/faq133.pdf?dmc=1&ts=20141102T2114483181

[8] Birth.com.au (2013). "Measuring and feeling your belly and listening to your baby". Retrieved from http://www.birth.com.au/tests-offered-during-pregnancy/feeling/measuring-your-belly-listening-to-baby#.VFbltfldWVM

[9] Csanyi, Carolyn (2013). "How to Hear Your Baby's Heartbeat With a Stethoscope" Retrieved from http://www.ehow.com/how_6954670_hear-baby-s-heartbeat-stethoscope.html.

[10] Cain, Candice (2013). "How to Detect a Fetal Heartbeat on Doppler" Retrieved from http://www.ehow.com/how_2363481_detect-fetal-heartbeat-doppler.html.

[11] Lucile Packard Children's Hospital (2013). "Common Tests During Pregnancy." Retrieved from http://www.lpch.org/DiseaseHealthInfo/HealthLibrary/pregnant/tests.html.

[12] Oladapo OT. "Amniocentesis and chorionic villus sampling for prenatal diagnosis: RHL commentary (last revised: 1 April 2009)." *The WHO Reproductive Health Library*; Geneva: World Health Organization. Retrieved from http://apps.who.int/rhl/pregnancy_childbirth/fetal_disorders/prenatal_diagnosis/CD003252_Oladapot_com/en/.

[13] Buckley, Sarah (2005). "Ultrasound Scans – Cause for Concern." Retrieved from http://sarahbuckley.com/ultrasound-scans-cause-for-concern.

[14] U.S. Food and Drug Administration (2014). "Ultrasound Imaging". Retrieved from http://www.fda.gov/Radiation-EmittingProducts/RadiationEmittingProductsandProcedures/MedicalImaging/ucm115357.htm.

[15] U.S. Food and Drug Administration (2014). "Ultrasound Imaging". Retrieved from http://www.fda.gov/Radiation-EmittingProducts/RadiationEmittingProductsandProcedures/MedicalImaging/ucm115357.htm.

[16] Buckley, Sarah (2005). "Ultrasound Scans – Cause for Concern." Retrieved from http://sarahbuckley.com/ultrasound-scans-cause-for-concern.

[17] Wagner (1999). "Ultrasound: More Harm than Good?" Retrieved from http://www.midwiferytoday.com/articles/ultrasoundwagner.asp.

[18] Kresser (2011). "Natural childbirth IIb: ultrasound not as safe as commonly thought." Retrieved from http://chriskresser.com/natural-childbirth-iib-ultrasound-not-as-safe-as-commonly-thought.

[19] Centers for Disease Control and Prevention (2014). Group B Strep. Retrieved from http://www.cdc.gov/groupbstrep/about/prevention.html.

[20] Home Birth Reference Site (n.d.). "Group B Strep and Home Birth." Retrieved from http://www.homebirth.org.uk/gbs.htm.

[21] The Center for Unhindered Living (2006). "Do-It-Yourself Prenatal Care." Retrieved from http://www.unhinderedliving.com/prenatal.html.

[22] WebMD (2014). "Anemia in Pregnancy." Retrieved from http://www.webmd.com/baby/guide/anemia-in-pregnancy?page=1.

[23] Baby Center L.L.C. (2013) "Frequent urination during pregnancy." Retrieved from http://www.babycenter.com/0_frequent-urination-during-pregnancy_237.bc.

[24] Office on Women's Health (2012). "Urinary tract infection fact sheet." Retrieved from http://womenshealth.gov/publications/our-publications/fact-sheet/urinary-tract-infection.html#b.

[25] American Pregnancy Association (2014). "Bleeding During Pregnancy." Retrieved from http://americanpregnancy.org/pregnancycomplications/bleedingduringpreg.html.

[26] Mayo Clinic (2014). "Gestational Diabetes – Complications." Retrieved from http://www.mayoclinic.org/diseases-conditions/gestational-diabetes/basics/complications/con-20014854.

[27] Home Birth Reference Site (n.d.). "Group B Strep and Home Birth." Retrieved from http://www.homebirth.org.uk/gbs.htm.

[28] Home Birth Reference Site (n.d.). "Group B Strep and Home Birth." Retrieved from http://www.homebirth.org.uk/gbs.htm.

[29] Centers for Disease Control and Prevention (2012). "ABCs Report: Group B *Streptococcus*, 2012." Retrieved from http://www.cdc.gov/abcs/reports-findings/survreports/gbs12.html

[30] Harms, Roger W., M.D. (2011). "What can I do to treat hemorrhoids during pregnancy?" Retrieved from http://www.mayoclinic.org/healthy-living/pregnancy-week-by-week/expert-answers/hemorrhoids-during-pregnancy/faq-20058149.

[31] Mayo Clinic (2011). "Preeclampsia – Risk Factors." Retrieved from http://www.mayoclinic.org/diseases-conditions/preeclampsia/basics/risk-factors/con-20031644.

[32] Mayo Clinic (2014). "High blood pressure and pregnancy: Know the facts". Retrieved from http://www.mayoclinic.org/healthy-lifestyle/pregnancy-week-by-week/in-depth/pregnancy/art-20046098

[33] Mayo Clinic (2014). "High blood pressure and pregnancy: Know the facts". Retrieved from http://www.mayoclinic.org/healthy-lifestyle/pregnancy-week-by-week/in-depth/pregnancy/art-20046098

[34] Goldberg, Carey (2013). "Tragically Wrong: When Good Early Pregnancies Are Misdiagnosed As Bad." Retrieved from http://commonhealth.wbur.org/2013/10/ectopic-pregnancy-misdiagnosed-methotrexate

[35] Beech, Beverly Lawrence (1999).Ultrasound: Weighing the Propaganda Against the Facts. Originally Appeared in Midwifery Today Issue 51, Autumn 1999. Retrieved from http://www.midwiferytoday.com/articles/ultrasound.asp.

[36] American Pregnancy Association (2014). "Rh Factor." Retrieved from http://americanpregnancy.org/pregnancycomplications/rhfactor-2.html.

[37] American College of Obstetricians and Gynecologists (2013). "The Rh Factor: How It Can Affect Your Pregnancy." Retrieved from http://www.acog.org/~/media/For%20Patients/faq027.pdf?dmc=1&ts=20140524T1411580129.

[38] National Heart, Lung, and Blood Institute (n.d.). "What Is Iron-Deficiency Anemia?" Retrieved from http://www.nhlbi.nih.gov/health/health-topics/topics/ida/printall-index.html

[39] Mathur, Ruchi, MD, FRCP(C) (2014). "Hypothyroidism During Pregnancy (Thyroid Deficiency During Pregnancy)." Retrieved from http://www.medicinenet.com/hypothyroidism_during_pregnancy/article.htm

Chapter 3
Labor

Homebirth Prep-List

You don't need any special supplies to give birth. All you really need is a mother in labor, but it doesn't hurt to prepare a few additional items. I compiled a list of homebirth supplies to you get started. Some you probably have at home. Some you can find substitutes for. For peace of mind, it's a good idea to have everything ready by the time your baby is full-term, which happens at 36 or 37 weeks.

Tarp (to cover the flooring, especially carpet)

If you're not worried about your floors, because they're old or clean up easily, you don't have to get a tarp. Otherwise, a suitable tarp found in the camping or painting section of your local hardware store will make cleanup a breeze.

Old comforters (to put over the tarp to make it more comfortable for you)

You can get old comforters at a yard sale or second-hand store if you don't have any.

Mattress protector for your bed

If you don't already have a mattress protector, I highly recommend you get one. They're nice to have, especially if you plan on co-sleeping with your little one.

Old set of sheets for your bed

If you can't find old sheets for your bed, treat yourself to a new set and use your existing sheets. If you use enough pads on your bed or end up giving birth on the floor or in the tub, your sheets might stay clean for now.

Flexible straws (optional)

Purchase flexible straws to help you stay hydrated during labor and birth. If you're laboring in a tub, it's easier to drink from a straw than picking up a cup or a bottle.

Pads (big ones to put under you and menstrual pads)

Purchase extra-large pads to protect your bedding. You'll also need regular menstrual pads to use postpartum. The heavy bleeding should subside quickly, but postpartum bleeding can last for several weeks.

Hand-held mirror (to help you see your baby being born)

A hand-held mirror allows you to see what's going on during the birth. You can watch your baby being born, and you can use it later to examine yourself for tears.

A clock or watch (to note time of birth)

Have a watch or phone nearby to keep track of time and record this momentous event. Keep pen and paper ready to write it down.

Towels (to rub baby down and keep him warm)

Whenever you watch an old movie where a baby is about to be born, all that seems to be needed is hot water and towels, lots of towels. Warm towels keep your baby warm, but your body heat is even more useful.

Hat for the baby (optional)

Most mothers can't wait to purchase a hat for their newborn baby, because they're plain adorable. Your baby doesn't need to wear a hat, unless you're taking him outside in freezing weather. Putting a hat on your baby doesn't help him regulate his own body temperature. A hat may interfere with bonding.[1] Have you ever smelled a newborn baby? This seemingly insignificant act of sniffing your baby's head connects you in more ways than one. A hat just gets in the way.

Sterilized medical scissors or knife

Unless you plan on having a lotus birth, you'll need something to cut the umbilical cord. Fortunately, there's no need to hurry. Simply boil a pair of scissors (to sterilize them) whenever you're ready. You can even purchase special umbilical cord scissors. Alternatively, use a sterilized knife or hold a cord burning.

Clamp for the umbilical cord

Wait until the cord is limp and pale, allowing your baby to get most of his blood from the placenta. Use an umbilical cord clamp or ring or dental tape to tie off the umbilical cord. Sterilized shoestring is an excellent substitute. If you wait long enough, there won't be much blood and you can skip clamping the cord altogether.

Baby thermometer

Checking your newborn's temperature regularly throughout the first couple of days is a simple way to catch potential problems early. While you can probably tell if your baby develops a fever by touching or kissing his forehead, a thermometer will give you an idea of how serious it is. Remember temperature readings vary depending on where you're measuring (underarm, oral, or rectal).

Newborn diapers

You may want to invest in a small pack of disposable diapers just for the first few days. Cloth diapers are much better in the long run—I'm a fan myself. But disposables are often smaller and easier to fold, which is nice while you still have to be careful with the umbilical cord stump. You may be more concerned about stains in the diapers from meconium than the umbilical cord, but many parents report meconium washes out and doesn't stain. Others prefer to use liners until this stage has passed to make cleanup easier.

Peri bottle (small squirt bottle)

A Peri bottle is just a small squirt bottle you fill with warm water. It may be your lifesaver during the postpartum period. Even if you don't tear or only tear slightly, you may feel a little sore, especially when you urinate. Simply use the bottle to squirt water over your perineum before, during, and after urination for instant pain relief.

Tape Measure

You'll need to know how big your baby is for the birth certificate. It's difficult to measure an infant, because they like to curl up. Therefore, your measurements may vary slightly each time, but you can get a good estimate. The best tape measures for this purpose are the ones used for sewing.

Scale

A normal scale isn't accurate enough to weigh a newborn baby, but weighing your baby is a simple way to evaluate him and chart his growth. And while your baby may lose some weight in the first few days, he should be back to his birth weight in about two weeks after the birth. You can find new and used infant scales online.

Container for placenta (optional)

If you want to keep your placenta (to eat, examine, show to your neighbors, or grind up into a smoothie), have a container or a bowl ready for it.

Black trash bag

You may already have big trash bags at home, but keeping one aside to use for cleanup after the birth is probably not a bad idea. Anything disposable and soiled can go in here. Naturally, I recommend you delegate this task to your partner.

Nursing Bras

While there's some debate on the necessity of wearing a bra at all, most modern women wear one every day. It may be a good idea to buy a few nursing bras to contain leaks. While your milk won't come in until a day or two after the birth, you probably won't feel like going shopping for bras then. You can switch to nursing bras during your pregnancy if you want. If your (regular or nursing) bras don't fit well as your belly is growing, you can get a bra extender.

Nursing Pads

Even the best nursing bra won't absorb all the extra milk your breasts release before, during, and after nursing sessions. Keep a few nursing pads handy, just in case. You can buy reusable nursing pads made of cotton. However, cotton nursing pads aren't usually machine-washable nor can they go into the dryer. Therefore, you need to get enough extras to allow for drying time.

Cold and hot packs

Placing a cold pack on your engorged breasts will make them feel better without messing up your milk production. If you pump too much milk to reduce the pressure, your breasts will produce even more. It should only take a few days for your breasts to adjust.

Hot packs are helpful for any other pain you may experience, including cramps and back pain. Applying heat to the painful area will give you some relief.

Ibuprofen

Most households already have Ibuprofen. It's certainly possible to go without pain medication after giving birth. However, afterpains are often worse with the second and each subsequent child. Don't take more than the recommended dosage and don't take it too often. If the pain doesn't significantly lessen with Ibuprofen or get better in a few days, consult a doctor to rule out any serious problems. Instead of Ibuprofen, you can try herbal remedies. With herbal remedies, be just as careful about dosage because they can also be very potent and potentially harmful if used incorrectly.

Warm wash cloth / oil compress

Perineal support during labor can prevent tearing. You can use a warm compress on your perineum, while providing some counter-pressure during the pushing stage. You can make a compress the following way: Use an old washcloth or a piece of flannel and put it in cold-pressed castor oil. Next, wring out the cloth and put it on your perineum, then cover it with something waterproof. You can put a heating pad on top if you like. Alternatively, you can use a warm washcloth and press it against your perineum as you're giving birth.[2]

Prep-List Summary

- ☐ Tarp
- ☐ Old comforters
- ☐ Mattress protector
- ☐ Old sheet set
- ☐ Flexible straws (optional)
- ☐ Pads
- ☐ Hand-held mirror
- ☐ A clock or watch
- ☐ Towels
- ☐ Sterilized medical scissors or knife
- ☐ Umbilical cord clamp or ring/dental tape/string
- ☐ Baby thermometer
- ☐ Scale
- ☐ Camera
- ☐ Newborn diapers
- ☐ Peri bottle (small squirt bottle)
- ☐ Tape measure
- ☐ Container for placenta (optional)
- ☐ Large trash bag
- ☐ Nursing bras
- ☐ Nursing pads
- ☐ Cold/Hot packs
- ☐ Ibuprofen
- ☐ Birthing Cheat Sheet printout
- ☐ Pen
- ☐ Warm wash cloth/Oil compress
- ☐ _____
- ☐ _____
- ☐ _____
- ☐ _____

Are You Really in Labor?

Whether this is your first or tenth baby, you may not be sure if you're experiencing true labor symptoms. I have some good news and some bad news for you. Many signs suggest labor is near, and your body is getting ready to give birth. Unfortunately, none of those signs are clear-cut.

For example, you may have contractions, but birth could still be a few weeks away. Personally, I found this rather difficult to cope with, especially at the end of my pregnancy. Every woman is different. You probably won't notice all the possible signs of labor, and you certainly shouldn't set the clock by any of them.

If you've never had a baby before, you may be nervous you won't recognize when you're in true labor. And while some women just pop out their babies, that's certainly not the norm. If you are one of those women who have their babies on the toilet without realizing they're in labor, you can count yourself lucky. There's no need to worry, because labor will be easy and spontaneous. Chances are you'll notice long before your baby starts crowning. And I'm here to help you familiarize yourself with the signs of labor.

Recognizing when you're in labor is helpful, because it allows you to prepare. However, labor lasts for a while. You don't need to alert too many people right away, especially if you don't want to be bothered by them.

The following list of labor symptoms is organized alphabetically, because signs of labor don't occur in a specific order, and you may not notice some of them at all.

(Recurring) Back Pain

If you experience recurring back pain, you might have contractions. Many women can feel contractions in their back first. This is also known as back labor. If the pain comes and goes and gets stronger, you may be in labor. Most pregnant women will have back pain at some point or another, especially during the third trimester. However, recurring lower back pain that radiates to the front might signal the beginning of labor.

As with any back pain, find a comfortable position to be in. The pain may go away, but it may get stronger if your baby has determined this is the day. Either way, do whatever makes you feel better. For example, you can lie on your side, use a hot pillow, get a massage from your partner, or pace the hallway. You can even take a warm bath, but please have someone help you get in and out of the tub to prevent a slip-and-fall accident.

Bloody Show / Mucous Plug

As the name "bloody show" entails, there may be some light bleeding after you lose your mucous plug. The mucous plug closes the cervix during the nine months of your pregnancy. It may come out a week or two before your baby's birth, but it may happen during labor.

Contrary to its name, the mucous plug doesn't really look like a plug. It doesn't always come out in one piece, either. Instead, you might notice slimy, stringy, blood-tinged mucous a few weeks, days, or hours before the birth of your baby.[3] The bleeding shouldn't be heavy bleeding, but it might be comparable to the first day of your period. By the way, some women never notice the loss of their mucous plug at all, and it's nothing to worry about.

Contractions

Labor contractions can start as pains in your lower back that move to the front of the abdomen. Pre-labor contractions—which do not result in your baby being born that day—are sometimes felt in your abdomen only. They may feel more like menstrual cramps than contractions.

Some women experience contractions in their back or legs, others only feel them in the front. Every labor is different. Where contractions are felt also depends on the position of the baby.

Your contractions have a purpose. When your uterus contracts, it helps open your cervix. Your cervix has to be completely opened (dilated) to about 10 cm for your baby to be born. Therefore, contractions are necessary for labor to progress. You may even have contractions a few weeks before your baby is born. If this is your first baby, you might not have any "practice contractions" until you go into labor. Oftentimes, actual labor may last longer for a first-time mother.

To clarify, contractions not part of active labor are commonly referred to as Braxton-Hicks contractions or false labor. While they may not lead to the birth of your baby *today*, they still prepare your body for labor and get your cervix ready. With second and subsequent babies, this process may just happen in spurts. Your actual labor can be shorter with your second or third child, because your body has been working hard for a few weeks beforehand with more frequent Braxton-Hicks contractions.

When you're in active labor, your contractions will become stronger and more frequent. Unlike Braxton-Hicks contractions, true labor contractions don't diminish or go away when you change positions or activities. They tend to establish a pattern and increase in intensity and frequency.

When you experience contractions, whether or not they signal true labor, do whatever it takes to make yourself comfortable. If you want to pace the hallway, do so. But if you'd rather lie down and take a nap, do that instead. Sometimes, moving around or changing positions can lessen the pain you experience during the contractions. If your contractions stay irregular, or just come and go every so often, it may still take a while until your baby comes. On the bright side, at least you know your body is doing some hard work ahead of time.

The timing of the contractions is not necessarily the best indicator of how much longer labor will last, although contractions usually increase in duration and in frequency as labor progresses. The best indicator of progress is the increasing intensity of your contractions.

Diarrhea

You may experience diarrhea during the last few weeks or days of your pregnancy, or you may not have any loose stools until you're actually in labor. Diarrhea before and during labor is believed to clean out your passages for the baby. Even if you had diarrhea before and during labor, you may still have a bowel movement while you're pushing out your baby. This is totally normal, because there will be an enormous amount of pressure on your pelvic region. Whenever you experience diarrhea, make sure to stay hydrated.

Effacement and Dilation of the Cervix

With regular prenatal care, your doctor or midwife may check your cervix as you get closer to your due date. You may be 3 centimeters dilated and 70% effaced, but this doesn't mean you'll have your baby today.

Effacement describes the thinning of the cervix and is expressed in percentages. Your cervix gradually thins out (effaces) and opens up (dilates). The dilation is expressed in centimeters. At 10 centimeters, the cervix is considered fully dilated, and you'll enter the pushing stage.

Whether or not you're doing your own prenatal care, you really don't need to worry about checking your cervix. As described above, both dilation and effacement are poor indicators of when exactly labor is going to start or how much longer labor will last. For example, you can be dilated a few centimeters for several weeks. During labor, measuring effacement or dilation won't even help determine whether labor is moving along at a good pace. Significant progress of dilation and effacement can happen slowly over a period of several weeks or quickly within an hour. There's no way to know which end of the spectrum you're on by taking measurements.

A vaginal exam is required to check both effacement and dilation. As you've already learned in a previous chapter, a vaginal exam can be another unnecessary intervention. If you absolutely want to check your cervix at home, you'll need someone else to do this for you. But if you let your partner check you, you might not be any wiser afterwards. It takes lots of practice, because you can only use your fingers to determine effacement and dilation of the cervix. The risk of him hurting you or accidentally breaking your water is significantly higher for a layperson than for a trained midwife, doula, or doctor.

Lightening

Lightening during pregnancy describes the descent of your baby into your pelvis. You'll probably be able to feel your baby has dropped. There is increased pressure on your bladder, and you might take up permanent camp in the bathroom. But you may breathe a little easier now since your baby has moved away from your lungs. If you've been struggling with heartburn, lightening might bring some relief from that as well. When you're having your first baby, lightening can occur several weeks before the birth, but if this is your second or subsequent baby, he may not drop until you're already in labor.

Nesting

Nesting is a behavior recorded by many women in their last trimester. As the time of birth approaches, they have this incredible urge to spring-clean and get their "nest" ready for the baby. You may not experience nesting at all, or you may stay up all night cleaning, because you just can't help it.

Nesting doesn't indicate labor is imminent. It can happen weeks or days before the birth of your baby. Nesting has some advantages.

Most women feel much better once their house is clean. This may be especially true for you if you're worried your partner won't keep up the housework while you're busy with your new baby. One reason for nesting: women know that nobody will do the chores while they're recovering from childbirth.

If you have an exceptionally strong nesting instinct and clean the same things twice, please drop by my house and continue cleaning any time. But if you want to do something more productive for yourself, cook and freeze a few extra meals. This will make life postpartum a little easier for you.

Water Breaking

In movies, a woman's water often breaks suddenly and leaves a huge puddle on the floor. She then barely makes it to the hospital to pop out the baby. As to be expected, real life is completely different.

Your water can "break" prior to labor, even prior to having any contractions. On the other extreme of the spectrum, your baby may be born with the bag of waters still intact. If this happens, you need to rupture the bag of waters manually after birth to allow your baby to breathe. Your water may break during labor or right before your baby is born.

Your water is the amniotic fluid in the sack surrounding your baby. When your water breaks, it may gush out or just trickle out. The liquid is normally clear and odorless. It's difficult to differentiate urine from amniotic fluid, because you may experience incontinence at the end of your pregnancy. Here are a few pointers to help you determine which of the two you're dealing with:

- Urine is at least slightly yellow.
- Urine has a distinctive smell.
- Amniotic fluid is odorless and clear.

- Amniotic fluid will trickle out constantly, but urine may not.[4]
- If you test the pH of the fluid, amniotic fluid will be alkaline, while urine is slightly acidic for most people.

If you determine your water has broken, there's no need to panic. If your water breaks before labor begins, contractions will most likely start within the next day or two.

Once your water is broken, there's an increased risk of infection. Therefore, if you don't go into labor soon, you need to check your temperature regularly. An elevated temperature signals an infection, and the fever is a sign your body is fighting it. If you develop a fever, you need to go to the hospital to induce labor.

Another reason to be concerned if your water breaks before labor: the amniotic fluid is green or brown instead of clear. This can signal that your baby is in distress (see the section about meconium-stained amniotic fluid below).

While most women will go into labor within 48 hours after the water has broken, some won't. According to Gloria Lemay, there are women who have gone six weeks with amniotic fluid leaking, giving birth to a healthy baby near their due date. She suggests women shouldn't be treated any differently, unless they develop a fever. However, if your water has broken, there should be no vaginal exams, and you need to refrain from sexual intercourse. Additionally, it's important to drink plenty of fluids, take showers instead of baths, and always wipe front to back on the toilet.[5] On a side note, she refers to the "breaking of the waters" as "membrane release", because there's really nothing broken about the process of childbirth.

A study evaluated the difference between waiting 12 and 72 hours for 566 women whose membranes had ruptured prematurely. "Fifty-five percent of the 12-hour group underwent oxytocin induction, compared with 17.5% of those in the 72-hour group".[6] Merely waiting an extra 2.5 days made an enormous difference in the induction rate without changing anything else. The findings state that waiting 12 or 72 hours was "comparable regarding infectious complications and pregnancy outcome". Therefore, there's no reason to induce labor immediately after your membranes have ruptured if there are no other concerns. Unfortunately, most doctors induce labor right away. Just beware, if you show up at the hospital after your water has broken without being in active labor, the medical personnel will induce you, even if you're not running a fever and it isn't medically necessary to rush the birth.

Meconium-Stained Amniotic Fluid

If your water breaks, the fluid should be clear and odorless (unlike urine, which has a strong smell to it). If your water is not clear but green or brown instead, then you may be concerned. Discolored amniotic fluid could be an indicator your baby is in distress, and it's no longer safe to continue the pregnancy.

I found an interesting article about meconium in the water. You may want to read it and come to your own conclusions. Rachel Reed states "meconium alone cannot be relied on as an indication of fetal distress."[7] According to a study of 4,026 births in 1991, "the cause of fetal distress and neonatal respiratory distress (RD) in association with meconium-stained liquor is not always clear."[8] In that study, 17.8% (717) of babies had meconium-stained waters, but only 1.2% (49) of babies developed respiratory distress. The study did not take into consideration how the babies were born and if interventions caused the fetal distress.

When meconium is found in the amniotic fluid, medical professionals are concerned your baby may have Meconium Aspiration Syndrome. First, understand this condition is rare, but it can be fatal. Fortunately, during a natural labor and birth, it's highly unlikely for your baby to inhale amniotic fluid with meconium in it, because babies rarely try to breathe until after they're born. However, if your baby becomes extremely hypoxic (a hypoxic baby is deprived of oxygen), she may gasp for air.

In her article, Reed reasons when meconium is found in the amniotic fluid, it's extremely important to prevent the baby from becoming hypoxic to avoid further complications. However, with meconium in the amniotic fluid, common practice is to do things known to cause hypoxia (for example, inducing labor, breaking the waters, directed pushing, having extra people in the room, cutting the cord early, and stressing the mother).

Reed suggests creating a relaxing birth environment and assuring the mother that meconium in the amniotic fluid is a variation, but not necessarily a complication.

Unfortunately, the risk of Meconium Aspiration Syndrome (MAS) is real. "The figure quoted for infants born with meconium-stained liquor in the industrialised world is 8-25% of births after 34 weeks of gestation. MAS occurs in around 1-3% of live births."[9] However, meconium may be present in the waters because of fetal distress or because your baby's gut has matured. Unfortunately, it's impossible to tell the difference between the two.

The important question now is what should you do if you discover meconium in your amniotic fluid? It depends. If labor is progressing rapidly and birth is imminent, you may not have time to transfer. If other indications show your baby is fine, you may decide to leave well enough alone. But with meconium aspiration, your baby might need assistance after birth. Fortunately, with proper treatment, "nearly all infants with MAS have complete recovery of pulmonary function."[10] It's very important to evaluate your newborn immediately after birth to ensure he's not having any difficulties breathing.

I have some personal experience with meconium in the water. During the birth of my fifth child, my water broke shortly before she was born. The fluid was green instead of clear. In my case, there was no need to worry and no time to do anything but give birth as planned. Our daughter was born healthy, with meconium on her body and head, but without breathing problems.

Inducing Labor

Once you've reached and passed your due date, and often several weeks beforehand, you may be tired of being pregnant. Every month has at most 31 days, but the last month of pregnancy has about 4,532 days.

We usually consider babies to be full-term at 37 weeks. Most babies are born between 38 and 42 weeks. But for some reason, your due date is set at 40 weeks.

In reality, nobody knows exactly when your baby is ready to be born. You'll probably be ready before him, and as time goes on, waiting for the big day may become difficult. Then you might look up symptoms of labor to find some in yourself. Unfortunately, knowing the signs of labor is usually no help at all.

Next thing you know, you might consider a natural induction method a friend told you about. Why not try it, since it worked for her, right? Before you go out and buy castor oil, bear with me for a couple more pages.

Women who choose to give birth at a hospital with a doctor in attendance will probably be induced with Pitocin before they get too far along. Some doctors even induce labor on an elective basis before the due date, just because the woman doesn't want to be pregnant anymore. I find this highly suspect. Here's why:

Due dates are inaccurate, even if you know the date of conception. Sperm can survive for a few days inside your body, and so can your unfertilized egg. If you don't know your conception date, you're relying on the first day of your last period to estimate when conception has taken place. This can vary widely.

And regardless of when your baby was conceived, some babies just take longer to "cook". It's not an exact science in which every woman's body produces a child in the exact same number of days. Naturally, gestation time varies, and that's why there's a range. It's the same for animals. And nobody will induce an elephant cow, just because she has gone past 22 months of gestation.

If you don't go into labor on your own, it's because your baby is not ready. No woman has ever stayed pregnant forever, and you certainly won't be the first one.

If you're past your "due date", I understand how anxious you are for labor to begin. I've been there myself. And since you're going to look up induction methods anyway, you might as well read about them here.

Experiences vary with induction methods. The placebo affect is likely involved—if you believe something will put you into labor, it just might. Do your research first, because having a healthy baby is goal number one. When the baby is born is not as important.

Induction Methods

If you want to establish an order of preference for induction methods, you might choose the least invasive options first, for example, walking or having sex. The last resort is using a drug like Pitocin. Here are the methods we'll discuss:

- Walking
- Sex
- Spicy foods
- Massage
- Primrose oil
- Castor oil
- Acupressure

- Acupuncture
- Nipple stimulation

Many people recommend walking to induce labor. Walking rocks your pelvis back and forth, which may help your baby position herself properly. If you're having contractions, walking may make them become stronger and more regular.

Of course, this only works if your body is ready. Don't expect walking around to make you go into labor. However, walking won't harm you, and it may distract you from being "overdue". You can walk as much as you want, as long as you don't over-exert yourself and stay hydrated.

Another way to induce labor naturally is to have sex with your partner. This may or may not sound like fun to you at this stage of your pregnancy. Sex can start labor because semen contains prostaglandins, which can stimulate your cervix.

If your body isn't ready to go into labor, having sex won't start it. But if your body just needs a little nudge, this may do it for you.

For me personally, sex didn't induce labor even after I passed 42 weeks of pregnancy (neither did castor oil). Other women reported more success. But as long as you have fun, there's no harm in trying. However, don't have sex after your water has broken, because you can risk an infection.

Spicy foods have a reputation of bringing on contractions by irritating your intestines, but to a lesser degree than castor oil. You may just end up with heartburn instead. If you normally eat spicy foods, there's probably nothing wrong with you continuing to do so. However, if you're used to eating spicy foods, I can't imagine how they would induce labor at any point.

Getting a massage can sometimes help a woman go into labor if her body is ready. There are two plausible explanations for this: One, the practitioner may have used the acupressure points (described soon). Two, getting a massage can raise your body's oxytocin levels, a hormone necessary for labor, because you're relaxed. The hormone oxytocin is also the reason labor often starts at night—that's when the mother is most relaxed.

Other commonly known induction methods listed next are not natural or intuitive. They can have harmful side effects, and none of them have been proven to induce labor reliably. Believe it or not, even Pitocin doesn't always induce labor. Sometimes, if your baby isn't ready, Pitocin won't get labor going. Unfortunately, a failed induction in a hospital setting will almost always lead to a C-section.[11]

In reality, a failed induction means your body works. If your baby had been ready to be born, you would have gone into labor on your own. Convincing doctors of this is futile.

While I don't recommend trying any of the following induction methods, I'm going to mention them just the same. Please think of your baby before you try any of them. Do you really want to kick him out early if he's not ready to be born?

Evening primrose oil is believed to get the cervix ready for labor.[12] There are other herbs, which may stimulate labor, but this herb is really not meant to induce. Midwives like evening primrose, because it's not believed to be harmful and can sometimes get labor going. You can get primrose oil capsules at almost every health-food store. Those capsules can be taken orally or inserted vaginally. If you decide to use them vaginally, you can puncture them before insertion, but they will dissolve on their own even if you don't puncture them. If you look up primrose oil on a site like herbwisdom.com, you may notice it's not recommended for pregnant or breastfeeding mothers.[13] You can probably find the same warnings on the bottle of castor oil.

Castor oil has long been rumored to start labor. It basically "works" by dehydrating your body and cleaning out your bowels, which may stimulate your uterus to contract. Besides the fact that castor oil is difficult to get down (it's disgusting—trust me), dehydrating your body is never a good idea. You can find castor oil in grocery stores, usually with other laxatives. The limited studies done on castor oil have found it to be neither harmful nor helpful with labor inductions[14].

My personal experience with castor oil is not encouraging. I felt desperate after 42 weeks and 3 days, and I took a tablespoon of castor oil. While it caused contractions and kept me on the toilet all night, labor didn't start because of it. I now completely understand why women try it at the end of pregnancy, but personally, I wouldn't do it again. My first unassisted baby was born at 43 weeks and 2 days without further meddling on my part. When I gave birth unassisted for the second time, I didn't try to induce labor at all and finally gave birth at 43 weeks and 6 days (my birth experiences are in the back of the book).

Acupuncture and acupressure are two other methods often used to induce labor. Acupuncture uses needles to stimulate certain pressure points in your body which are associated with uterine activity. Acupressure does the same thing, but without needles. Instead, acupressure uses pressure or massage. Don't try acupuncture at home unless your partner does this for a living. Acupressure is something you can technically do by yourself, or your partner can do it for you.

The idea behind acupressure is to use finger pressure on different areas of your body to induce labor. Two of these areas, which correspond to uterine activity, are the webbed area between your thumb and index finger, and the inside of your leg (four finger-widths above your anklebone).

"Use prolonged finger pressure directly on the point; gradual, steady, penetrating pressure for approximately three minutes is ideal."[15] As with any other induction method, women report various results. If your body is ready, acupressure may put it over the edge. However, it may not work for you at all.

Another induction method is nipple stimulation. If nipple stimulation is successful, it can cause powerful contractions. For this to work, you may require a breast pump. Merely playing with your nipples during sex won't make your body go into labor. However, contractions may start from vigorous sucking action on your nipples.

Some women have used nipple stimulation successfully after labor has stalled, to avoid other medical interventions. For example, labor may have stalled once they got to the hospital. To avoid Pitocin or a C-section, nipple stimulation may have helped many women have a natural birth. But when you give birth at home on your own, there's no need to resort to nipple stimulation. It's perfectly plausible for labor to take time. As long as both mother and baby are doing okay, it's probably better to just wait patiently.

Summing up, there are quite a few things you can do to give things a little nudge. But since none of them are guaranteed to work, the best advice is to relax and wait patiently for labor to begin naturally.

When You're Overdue

A "normal" pregnancy lasts between 38 and 42 weeks. It starts with the first day of your last menstrual cycle. Technically, during the first couple of weeks of pregnancy, you're not even pregnant yet. Conception usually happens two or three weeks afterwards. By the time you hold a positive test in your hand, you may already be considered five or six weeks along.

The due date is arbitrarily chosen as the 40-week mark, right in the middle, between 38 and 42 weeks. Do you see why the due date makes me so mad? It feels like you're late and overdue, when in reality, you still have two weeks where your baby is considered full-term. Only when you're still pregnant after 42 weeks is your pregnancy considered post-term.

The due date calculation is not an exact science, even if this is what medicine will have you believe. Due dates only came about in the 1950s. Before then, women had a due month, which is a much more accurate way of describing when birth is going to happen. You're not really past due until you go over 42 weeks, which isn't likely, according to statistics.

Of course, those statistics are skewed, because most doctors will induce a pregnant woman by 41 weeks. The average length of gestation would probably be higher if you sampled a group of women who didn't use any methods of induction.

Some women will actually give birth on their due date. Many women go past their due date, especially if it's their first child. Therefore, a due date of 40 weeks really only gets peoples' hopes up inaccurately. Babies come when they're ready. Many times, women get induced only to have a rather small baby. This same baby could have used more time in the womb, which is precisely why labor hadn't started naturally.

A friend of mine went 15 days past her due date with her third baby. The ultrasound at 42 weeks revealed that her baby's abdomen was measuring small, and the doctor induced labor. The baby only weighed 7 pounds. She probably would have been just fine "cooking" a little longer, but doctors get nervous. A lot of doctors will schedule an induction at 41 weeks for no other reason than due-date anxiety.

Whenever people ask you about your "late" baby, simply reassure them you and your baby are healthy, and the best option is to continue the pregnancy until you go into labor naturally. Inducing has its own risks not necessarily worth taking. **Your baby will come when he is ready.**

If you go significantly past your due date, there may come a time when you break down and cry. Don't worry, this is completely normal. After all, you have unmet expectations. Throw in some pregnancy hormones, and a minor crisis or even a full-blown panic attack is not entirely unexpected.

When this happens, remember nobody has ever been pregnant forever. Treasure your pregnancy as much as you can and relax. If you need to, go into hiding and only talk to people who are supportive of your choices and avoid the rest of the population.

For specific concerns easily resolved with a simple check-up, you can schedule a prenatal appointment. For example, at the end of my pregnancy, I worried my baby wouldn't come, because he was traverse breech. A vaginal exam at 42 weeks revealed him to be heads down. After knowing this, I visibly relaxed and stressed less for the rest of my pregnancy. Nobody can induce you against your will, and you can even refuse further testing.

Post-Term Pregnancy

Inductions are risky. When inductions fail (and yes, they can fail), it means your body wasn't ready to go into labor. If you're getting induced at the hospital, and you don't go into labor, then you'll probably have a C-section. It doesn't sound like a good thing to me.

I don't understand why we can't just be patient and wait until the baby is ready to come. Elephants have to be pregnant for 22 months, and no one ever induces them when they go past their due date. Humans are the only species to forcefully end a pregnancy instead of letting the body take care of it.

Why Is a Post-Term Pregnancy a Problem?

The medical world claims post-term pregnancies can be a risk to both the mother and the baby. Most women are induced before they reach 42 or even 41 weeks of pregnancy.

According to a study on post-term pregnancies published by Facts Views Vis Obgyn (2012), the placenta deteriorates as the pregnancy continues. Doctors often worry about the amniotic fluid levels becoming insufficient for the baby. Finally, there is the concern your baby will get too big, and therefore, he won't fit through the birth canal.[16] The same study recommends labor to be induced by 41 weeks, because "postterm pregnancy is associated with fetal, neonatal and maternal complications including morbidity and perinatal mortality."[17]

The placenta nourished your baby throughout your entire pregnancy. It's absurd to think it would have an expiration date and stop functioning after exactly nine months. Obviously, once the baby is ready to be born, the placenta has accomplished its purpose. Who is to say labor and the end of the placenta's useful life don't go together, one causing the other?

The same thing might be true about the amniotic fluid. Who is to say it isn't normal and expected of fluid levels to change as pregnancy nears its end? The belief that your baby might not fit through the birth canal if your pregnancy lasts another week or two seems ridiculous as well.

Besides, doctors rely on ultrasound to determine the size of the baby. Ultrasound is notoriously wrong when estimating a baby's weight. Your body and your baby are unique. Every pregnancy is going to be unique. Your belly will look different with each pregnancy. For example, you may look huge and still give birth to a small baby. Or your belly may look small, but your baby is a little butterball.

Post-term pregnancies don't automatically end in big babies. Both of my post-term babies were average size. My first boy was born at 43 weeks and 2 days weighing 7 pounds 10 ounces. My second boy and second unassisted birth didn't happen until 43 weeks and 6 days gestation, but my baby only weighed 7 pounds 11 ounces. Clearly, they both needed the additional time in the womb.

With a post-term pregnancy, doctors are often concerned with the woman's physical ability to continue carrying a child. They worry about preeclampsia and a host of other things I will cover later. Doctors don't have faith in a woman's ability to give birth or a baby's ability to be born healthy. Their education is fear-based, and they're trained for complications. You'll have a hard time finding a doctor who's supportive of a post-term pregnancy, especially once you go past 42 weeks or even 43 weeks. Even the best midwives get nervous once you go past 42 weeks.

The American College of Obstetricians and Gynecologists (ACOG) issued the following guidelines for a post-term pregnancy in 2004: "Women with post-term gestations who have unfavorable cervixes can either undergo labor induction or be managed expectantly. Prostaglandin can be used in post-term pregnancies to promote cervical ripening and induce labor. Delivery should be affected if there is evidence of fetal compromise or oligohydramnios [low amniotic fluid levels]."[18]

In her article "Induction of Labour: Balancing Risks", Rachel Reed writes: "There is, in fact, no logical reason for believing that the placenta, which is a fetal organ, should age while the other fetal organs do not..."[19] She also observes there is some concern about the quality of the research done on post-term pregnancies. Even the World Health Organization acknowledges that the evidence is low-quality evidence. Yet they still recommend induction of labor by 41 weeks.

How to Cope

It's stressful if your friends and family members constantly ask you about your baby after you've passed your due date. You could assure them you'll keep them posted about the big event and ask them to leave you alone in the meantime. Waiting for a baby isn't easy under the best of circumstances. The longer it takes, the more difficult it becomes, and doubts can creep in.

When you find yourself in this situation, repeat this to yourself: your body really knows what to do. I promise. Your body will go into labor when your baby is ready. Please believe me and search for some uplifting stories. Women are catching on that going into labor on their own is natural, but picking your baby's birthday by getting induced is not.

During the end of your pregnancy, find things to do to distract yourself. At least once a day, plan an activity you need to leave the house for. Go window-shopping, go to a park, or eat some ice cream with a supportive friend. Stay away from people who are not supportive, because they will just add to your worries.

If you're harboring secret fears around the upcoming birth, resolve them as best as you can. If you're unsure of the baby's position, get it checked out. Your pregnancy symptoms won't differ from before only because you've passed 42 weeks. You'll feel tired, and you'll have spurts of energy. You may have more back pain, but it's natural since your baby is putting a lot of strain on your back.

Connect with other moms who've been there. Read something reassuring. It doesn't have to be related to childbirth, but it could be an inspirational book. Watching comedy can help, too. It's hard to see it now, but you'll miss being pregnant later. Therefore, relax and enjoy it a little bit.

What to Expect

Now that you're "past due", you can expect people to offer unsolicited advice or ask questions such as, "Is your doctor going to induce you?", or "Does your doctor think you'll go into labor soon?" People will advise you to get induced, because they heard it's not safe for the baby to stay in your womb past your due date.

Regardless of what people around you're saying, you'll go through some emotional turmoil as well. You'll feel like you've reached the end of your rope and that you can't stand it another day. You may give up hope and envision what it will be like to be pregnant forever. You may feel depressed and moody. You may have a nervous breakdown and cry your eyes out. There will be days where you wake up feeling great. As the day progresses, your mood might change again to the darker side. All of this is perfectly normal.

Your logical mind knows your baby will come, and that it's only a matter of time. And yet, it's difficult to keep the faith the longer it takes. You might even start thinking this was all just a dream, and you're not really pregnant at all. As silly as it seems, this happened to me, and I wasn't the only one. But don't worry, everything will be fine. You'll be fine, and your baby will be fine, and you'll have a good laugh about it later.

You still need to take good care of yourself by eating a nutritious diet and drinking plenty of water. Enjoy the last few days and weeks of your pregnancy. Think of all the things you won't be able to do once your baby shows up and try to do some of them. Sleep comes to mind.

Having a newborn baby will be wonderful, but being pregnant can be fun, too. Enjoy feeling your baby move around without having to share him and without having to soothe his crying. He will be here before you know it.

Why You Should Wait until Your Baby Is Ready

If you and your baby are healthy, there's absolutely no reason to rush him out. While there are some natural induction methods, many of them have potential side effects. Besides, inductions without health reasons are unnecessary. If your baby was ready, you would go into labor. That you're not in labor means she's not ready to be born yet.

Even though we know the average length of pregnancy, and we consider a baby born at 37 weeks full-term, we can never know exactly when your baby is fully developed. A baby born at 39 weeks may have breathing problems, and a baby born at 36 weeks might not. You never know. If you wait until you go into labor naturally, you can be pretty sure your baby is ready to be born.

If you agree to an induction at the hospital, you need to be aware of the risks associated with it. I have described them in my chapter on interventions, and I don't want to repeat the information here. Just know it's better to wait the baby out, unless there is a medical need for an induction. This is true whether you're 38, 41, or 43 weeks pregnant.

To be fair, inducing labor can end well. You may even give birth without an epidural, and your baby will most likely still turn out fine. But she would have preferred to stay in your womb a little longer, and it wouldn't have hurt either of you. The bottom line is inductions have their own sets of risks. Therefore, they shouldn't be performed routinely, just because a not-so-magical due date has passed.

Expectant Management

If you hired a doctor or a midwife, let them know you want to continue the pregnancy. As long as there are no indications of any problems, it's much safer to stay pregnant and wait until labor starts on its own. A doctor will probably insist on regular fetal stress tests, ultrasounds, or both, to monitor your baby. Again, it's your choice to decide how much prodding you want to endure. While it's certainly not harmful to check your baby's heartbeat with a stethoscope, using a fetal monitor for a fetal stress test can be (see my chapter on the dangers of interventions).

In conclusion, expectant management sounds like a good idea, but it may still lead to an induction without a legitimate reason. It's your choice to decide how much monitoring you want done. You know better than any doctor if there's something wrong if you pay attention to your body. If she is moving around as usual, everything is probably just fine.

What to Watch Out For

When you go past your due date or even exceed 42 weeks, nothing much changes. There are a few things you want to watch out for, because complications could be more likely at this point.

There should be regular fetal movements. Some women like to count kicks or movements within a certain timeframe, but you don't have to do that. If you can't feel your baby move at all, seek medical assistance. But before you panic and run to the hospital, try to get your baby to move by doing one or more of the following things:

- Drink something cold
- Eat something containing sugar
- Drink something with caffeine
- Change positions
- Walk around or lie down (depending on your previous activity—try the opposite)
- Feel for your baby by gently pressing along your belly

Have you ever noticed how your baby usually kicks and wiggles when you're trying to sleep? That's because he woke up. You're not moving around, and therefore, you aren't rocking him anymore. When you move around, the motion will put him to sleep. This works after birth, too. Most babies fall asleep in swings, strollers, cars, and when being carried and rocked.

If none of these techniques work, and you can't feel any movement, go to the nearest hospital. Hopefully, they'll reassure you all is well, and your baby is just having an awfully lazy day.

Another concern during late pregnancy is preeclampsia, which is pregnancy-induced high blood pressure. You need to look out for the following symptoms:

- Sudden swelling of your hands, feet, or face
- Sudden weight gain
- A severe headache that won't go away with Tylenol
- Severe pain in your stomach (not contractions)
- Vision changes (for example blurry vision, flashing lights, or temporary blindness)
- Vomiting
- Decreased urination

Preeclampsia often goes hand in hand with an unhealthy diet and limited exercise. To keep your blood pressure stable and your body and your baby healthy, eat plenty of fresh fruits and vegetables and drink lots of water while staying away from processed foods and drinks. If you can go for a walk—even a short one—it can make a big difference in how you feel.

Another concern at the end of pregnancy is your water breaking before you go into labor. If your water has broken, it will either gush out, or you'll notice a small trickle. After your water has broken, there's an increased risk of infection. Most often, labor will start within a few days after your water breaks. Until it does, check your temperature every few hours. If your temperature rises, and you develop a fever, it means your body's battling an infection. If this happens, you need to go to the hospital and have labor induced.

Finally, if you just don't feel right without being able to pinpoint why, please seek the advice of a medical professional. In most cases, pregnancy can continue until labor starts on its own, with no issues. But it's important to be aware of complications, which may arise (even though chances are small), because the number one goal is to ensure both mother and baby are safe.

Summary of Warning Signals

1. Your baby isn't moving
2. Sudden swelling of your hands, feet, and face

3. Sudden weight gain or loss
4. Severe headache that doesn't resolve with Tylenol
5. Severe pain in your stomach (not contractions)
6. Vision changes (such as blurriness)
7. Vomiting
8. Decreased urination
9. If you develop a fever after your water breaks
10. If you feel something is wrong

I want to encourage you to hang in there. I know it's really difficult, but if you wait just a little longer, you can have the birth of your dreams. In the meantime, talk to your baby and tell him how excited you are to finally meet him.

---

[1] "The Essential Homebirth Guide: For Families Planning or Considering Birth at Home" by Jane E. Drichta, Jodilyn Owen, and Dr. Christina Northrup

[2] Aasheim V, Nilsen ABVika, Lukasse M, Reinar LM. Perineal techniques during the second stage of labour for reducing perineal trauma. Cochrane Database of Systematic Reviews 2011, Issue 12. Art. No.: CD006672. DOI: 10.1002/14651858.CD006672.pub2.

[3] "The Essential Homebirth Guide: For Families Planning or Considering Birth at Home" by Jane E. Drichta, Jodilyn Owen, and Dr. Christina Northrup

[4] Murry, Mary M., R.N., C.N.M. (2010). "Rupture of membranes: Has your water broken?" Retrieved from http://www.mayoclinic.org/healthy-living/pregnancy-week-by-week/expert-blog/rupture-of-membranes/bgp-20055787.

[5] Lemay, Gloria (2008). "Membrane release before birth sensations begin, what to do?" Retrieved from http://wisewomanwayofbirth.com/membrane-release-before-birth-sensations-begin-what-to-do/.

[6] Comparison of 12- and 72-hour expectant management of premature rupture of membranes in term pregnancies. Obstet Gynecol. 1995 May ;85(5 Pt 1):766-8.

[7] Reed, Rachel (2010). The Curse of Meconium Stained Liquor. Retrieved from http://midwifethinking.com/2010/10/09/the-curse-of-meconium-stained-liquor/.

[8] Possible causes linking asphyxia, thick meconium and respiratory distress. Aust N Z J Obstet Gynaecol. 1991 May ;31(2):97-102.

[9] Louis D, Sundaram V, Mukhopadhyay K, et al; Predictors of mortality in neonates with meconium aspiration syndrome. Indian Pediatr. 2014 Aug 8;51(8):637-40.

[10] Dr Louise Newson (2014). Meconium-stained liquor. Retrieved from http://www.patient.co.uk/doctor/meconium-stained-liquor

[11] South Shore Medical Center (2014). "When your labor needs to be induced." Retrieved from http://www.ssmedcenter.com/healthy_pregnancy/labor_induced.cfm.

[12] JOSIE L. TENORE, M.D., S.M., "Methods for Cervical Ripening and Induction of Labor." *Am Fam Physician*. 2003 May 15;67(10):2123-2128. Retrieved from http://www.aafp.org/afp/2003/0515/p2123.html.

[13] Hallnet Ltd. (2014). "Evening Primrose Oil (Oenothera Biennis)." Retrieved from http://www.herbwisdom.com/herb-evening-primrose.html.

[14] U.S. National Library of Medicine "Castor oil for induction of labour: not harmful, not helpful". Aust N ZJ Obstet Gynaecol, 49(5), 499-503. Retrieved from https://obgyn.onlinelibrary.wiley.com/doi/abs/10.1111/j.1479-828X.2009.01055.x

[15] Michael Reed Gach, Ph.D. (2014). How to Apply Pressure to Acupressure Points. Retrieved from http://www.acupressure.com/articles/Applying_pressure_to_acupressure_points.htm.

[16] Galal, M., Symonds, I., Murray, H., Petraglia, F., Smith, R.. Postterm Pregnancy. Facts Views Vis Obgyn. 2012; 4(3): 175–187. Retrieved from http://www.ncbi.nlm.nih.gov/pmc/articles/PMC3991404/#.

[17] Galal, M., Symonds, I., Murray, H., Petraglia, F., Smith, R.. Postterm Pregnancy. Facts Views Vis Obgyn. 2012; 4(3): 175–187. Retrieved from http://www.ncbi.nlm.nih.gov/pmc/articles/PMC3991404/#.

[18] Neff, Matthew, J. (2004). ACOG Releases Guidelines on Management of Post-term Pregnancy

Retrieved from http://www.aafp.org/afp/2004/1201/p2221.html.

[19] Reed, Rachel (2014). Induction of Labour: balancing risks. Retrieved from http://midwifethinking.com/2010/09/16/induction-of-labour-balancing-risks/.

Chapter 4
Childbirth

Are Labor and Birth Painful?

First things first: pain is relative. Labor and childbirth may be painful if you expect them to be. Then again, you might be pleasantly surprised and experience only slight pains or none at all. Unfortunately, women in our society have been conditioned to believe being in labor and having a baby is unbearably painful, even to the point where pain relief is required.

Tribal women who give birth naturally don't harbor the same beliefs about childbirth. They know it's a natural process which doesn't require any intervention. Childbirth doesn't have to be painful. It can even be orgasmic for some women.[1] You can find books about orgasmic births, and if you think about it, it makes sense. Your uterus contracts when you have an orgasm. The same thing happens when you're in labor. Contractions in labor differ only in intensity.

Why do we feel pain during labor but not when we have an orgasm? We feel pain, because the intensity of the contractions is greater than we've ever experienced. We're also conditioned to believe labor and childbirth are painful.

Certain emotions can be counterproductive to enjoying the process. The biggest emotion you need to conquer is fear. Most "civilized people" are afraid of childbirth. We may not believe childbirth is the punishment for Eve's sins, but we still expect and fear pain. Whenever you're afraid, your body goes into its natural fight-or-flight response, during which oxygen is directed to your body, allowing you to either fight or run away. A person who's afraid will be white in the face, because the blood drains, enabling your legs to run. All non-essential body parts will be deprived of oxygen during this time.

Your uterus is one of those body parts considered non-essential in a fight-or-flight situation. And this makes sense, because if you were truly in danger and had to fight or flee, you wouldn't want labor to continue. Therefore, the uterus is deprived of oxygen when you're afraid, literally turning it white. Then it has no fuel, and this will make labor more difficult and more painful for you. If you want to learn more about this phenomenon, read "Childbirth without Fear" by Dr. Grantly Dick-Read. He's credited to have first discovered this reaction of the uterus to fear.

Other emotions contributing to feeling pain include shame and guilt. Many of us are not in tune with our bodies anymore. We cover up everywhere. When you give birth at the hospital, you get to wear a gown. At home, you would most likely have the urge to shed your clothes, which allows you to hold your baby skin-to-skin immediately after birth.

Besides being ashamed of our naked bodies, we are ashamed of their natural functions. As adults, we neither pee nor poop in front of other people, nor do we have sex in public. Elimination and sex are still natural behaviors, but they're private. It's not surprising giving birth is no different in that aspect. We are much more comfortable laboring and birthing in the privacy of our own homes than under the bright lights of a hospital room, surrounded by strangers.

So which emotions would be helpful for a laboring woman? You need to have faith in yourself and in your body. Be patient and loving with yourself and others. You must have the courage to stand up for what you believe in. Even if you end up having your baby at a hospital, you're the one who gets to decide what will be done. Doctors or nurses may not make it sound as if there's a choice, but you have the right to veto.

How to Cope with Labor Pains

During labor, you may find natural pain relief through the following methods:

- Meditation
- Hot or cold packs
- Getting a massage
- Bouncing on a birth ball
- Changing positions
- Taking a bath
- Guided imagery

If you don't already have a hot pillow, you can make your own using cloth and *uncooked* white rice. Since this takes a while and requires a needle and thread (or a sewing machine), don't wait until you go into labor to fashion one of these. The pillow is going to be a lot smaller than a regular pillow, but it should be a little longer than the width of your back. This will allow you to apply heat evenly when you need it. The pillow needs to be small enough to fit in the microwave.

How women cope with labor pains is uniquely up to each individual. Most women who give birth naturally find it helpful to rest as much as possible. Some enjoy their loved one(s) nearby, others prefer to be alone. You might like music or candlelight, or you might like to just curl up in bed. And as much as you can plan for eventualities by having everything available ahead of time, you may need none of it when the time comes, because your experience will probably differ from your expectations.

If you're unsure of what to expect in terms of pain during labor, it may help to read some birth stories or watch a few homebirth videos. Familiarize yourself with the process. I know you can do this and have the birth of your dreams, even if you sometimes doubt yourself along the way.

For many women, there comes a point during labor when they really want to give up. The contractions become intense, and you just can't stand it anymore. This is actually a sign you've reached transition, and this mean you're really close to having your baby.

How to Have a Water Birth

Most regular bathtubs aren't deep enough to allow you to submerse yourself into the water. If the idea of a water birth appeals to you, you can rent or purchase a birth pool ahead of time. If you can't find an affordable birth pool, a regular blow-up pool might work, too.

A water birth is often referred to as the midwife's epidural. You can stay in the tub for as long as it feels comfortable to you. When the water gets cold, have your partner add a pot of hot water. But the water temperature should stay around 96-98 degrees.

With a water birth, you need to follow a few safety rules. Obviously, you can't allow your baby to stay submerged under water after he's born. **You must bring the baby up out of the water immediately.** Otherwise, he will risk brain injury from lack of oxygen. If your baby swallows some water, he may have electrolyte problems. Finally, there is a risk of infection for you and your baby if the bath water is contaminated.[2]

Sometimes, a water birth is not advisable. For example, if your water has broken or you have an infection or herpes, giving birth on land is safer. But these concerns and risks aside, a lot of women simply swear by their water birth, knowing it was the best choice for them.

Since a water birth can reduce the need for pain medication and allow the woman to continue to labor naturally, there are a lot of benefits to giving birth in the water. And while many hospitals offer water births, not all of them will let you give birth in the water. In fact, they may require you to get out when it's time to have a baby. This is often contrary to the laboring woman's wishes. If you get into the tub for pain relief at home, then you probably won't want to get out for the birth.

Some people argue that giving birth in the water is unnatural since we aren't fish and can't live underwater. The only land mammals that give birth in the water are hippos, but hippos are equally comfortable in water and on land. The newborn hippo has to swim up to the surface to catch its first breath, but baby hippos even nurse underwater.

Tribal women rarely have water births. There are probably at least three reasons for this: One, they may not have access to clean water. Two, they don't need the water for pain relief. And finally, giving birth in the water requires assistance by another person to ensure the baby is lifted out of the water quickly.

I'm not against water births, but they're not my personal favorite. I gave birth to my second child in the water. But whether it was the tub, that I still labored in an unfavorable semi-reclined sitting position, the midwife's role in the birth, or something entirely different, I didn't have the desire to repeat my water birth. My three unassisted births all happened on land.

Being submerged in water is soothing and relaxes the mother while relieving the pain. You may be less likely to tear during the birth if you're in the water, although your position plays an even bigger role in keeping your perineum intact. Finally, water births have been shown to reduce the use of pain medication and other interventions. Of course, these aren't available when you give birth at home. But a water birth at the hospital can increase your chance of having a natural birth in that setting, too.

The only downside to a water birth is the need to plan for it. You'll need help in setting up the birth pool before you go into labor. If you live in a small place, there may be space issues to solve. Since labor can last for a while, the water will probably get cold before you want to get out. You'll need someone to add additional hot water to it. The water temperature should be around 97 degrees, although some sources say it can be up to 100 degrees. And even though you're submerged in water, you still need to stay hydrated by drinking plenty of fluids.

If you want to give birth in water at home, you absolutely can. But you don't have to. Follow your instincts and do some research. Even if you don't have a birth pool, getting into a regular tub might offer some relief during labor. Take advantage of it if you want, but don't feel pressured to give birth in the water, because it's the popular thing to do.

The 3 Stages of Labor

Labor is divided into three stages. While you don't have to notice each individual stage as you're going through it, it helps to have a general idea of how labor is going to progress. Just know that a natural labor and birth take time. Babies don't just pop out, despite what is often falsely portrayed in movies.

First Stage: Dilation of the cervix

Early Labor: dilation from 0 to 3 cm

Active Labor: dilation up to 7 cm

Transition: dilation up to 10 cm

Second Stage: Birth of your baby

Third Stage: Arrival of the placenta[3]

First Stage: Early Labor

Your cervix is in the lower portion of your uterus. When you're not pregnant, the cervix allows your menstrual blood to flow out. During pregnancy, the cervix stays closed and only opens to let your baby through for childbirth. The first stage of labor is the time between the on-set of true labor until your cervix is dilated up to 10 centimeters.

As you may already know, the first stage of labor takes the longest. It's usually subdivided into its own three phases: early labor, active labor, and transition. Physicians measure early labor to last until your cervix is dilated to 3 cm, active labor up to 7 cm, and transition until your cervix reaches 10 cm.

During early labor, you can still perform normal activities, as this is usually not too painful. Rest as much as you can during this time. If it's nighttime, try to get some sleep. Otherwise, do something you enjoy, such as reading a book or watching a movie. You'll need all of your energy later. Now's not the time to clean the house. If the mess really bothers you, make your partner take care of it.

Technically, early labor can last anywhere from a few hours to several weeks, with contractions coming and going sporadically. Some women, especially with second and subsequent pregnancies, will experience "practice" contractions. These may seem like labor but fizzle out and stop after a while, only to start up again days later. These contractions are Braxton-Hicks contractions or false labor. If you're full-term (past 37 weeks), there's usually nothing to worry about.

Personally, I don't like calling it false labor, because to your body it's not false. These preliminary contractions serve a purpose and get your body ready for the birth. However, you may not be sure whether it's the real thing, and this can be unnerving.

Early Labor To-Do List

Once you know you're in labor, you can look at your early labor to-do list. You can either get these things ready yourself or ask your partner to help you.

- Sterilize scissors, shoestring, etc.
- Put towels in the dryer
- Have a clock or watch ready
- Set up timer or stopwatch for checking baby's pulse
- Set up birthing area
- Put Peri bottle in the bathroom
- Make the bed

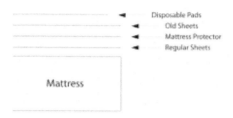

You(r partner) can make the bed the following way: Keep your regular sheets on your bed. Then put the mattress protector on top. On top of it, put a set of old sheets (flat sheets might make this easier). Last, line up some big disposable pads.

After the birth, your partner can take off the top layers and clean/dispose of them. This method helps immensely with cleanup. And your bed will quickly be ready for you to rest in with your baby.

First Stage: Active Labor

As you enter active labor, relaxing won't be easy. You may even feel like pacing the house or going for a walk. Follow your instincts. If you feel like walking, do so. Take your partner with you and lean on him when you need to. Your contractions will probably follow a pattern and increase in frequency and intensity.

Active labor can take a long time. Fortunately, every contraction brings you closer to your baby. If you're giving birth with a midwife or doctor, they may check your dilation periodically to assess your progress. And while it's nice to know how far your cervix has dilated, you still won't know how much longer it will take. Dilation can happen quickly or slowly, and there's no need to check it during an unassisted birth.

There are other, less-invasive ways to check on your progress. For one, your contractions will get stronger and more intense. They will increase in frequency as labor progresses. A skilled midwife would notice your behavior changing. A woman in early labor can still hold a conversation during a contraction, but during active labor or transition, this may not be possible.[4]

Every woman handles labor differently. Some want to be alone, some like having company, others might want to listen to music or watch TV. Do whatever you feel like doing at the moment. And don't forget to keep drinking and going to the bathroom regularly.

Don't worry about recognizing the phases of the first stage of labor. It's not necessary to differentiate between early labor, active labor, and transition to give birth successfully. Nobody can predict how long your labor will last, anyway. Just focus on the moment and do what feels right to you.

First Stage: Transition

During transition, when things are getting closer to the end, you'll probably feel the most pain. This is the point where women at the hospital might beg for pain relief. But in my humble opinion, this means it's time to have a baby and not an epidural.

It's natural to have moments of self-doubt during this time. Just keep breathing, because you can do this. It's like running a marathon: at the end, you get really worn out, but you don't want to give up if you can see the finish line. Once it's over, you'll feel great and proud of yourself, and the pain will be a distant memory.

While being familiar with meditation or other relaxation methods can help a woman during labor to stay calm, it's not a requirement for a natural birth. I hadn't meditated or practiced any other special relaxation or breathing techniques before giving birth, but when it was time to have a baby, my body automatically responded. As the intensity of the contractions increased, my breathing became deep and calm without conscious effort. If you want to meditate or look into breathing techniques, go for it. But you don't have to take a course on breathing to give birth, because you've been doing this since you were born. However, when it comes to breathing, keep these things in mind:

- Never hold your breath!
- Don't hyperventilate!

Stay calm and keep breathing. You may envision your baby descending into the birth canal with each wave. Knowing every contraction brings your baby closer to you is a lot more helpful than focusing on the painful sensations. Listen to your body and do what it tells you to do.

Your partner can massage you, you can listen to your favorite music, or you can pray, if you're so inclined. You may prefer to be left alone. A lot of women enjoy getting into the tub during transition. The warm water is especially soothing for a woman in labor. And if it's at all possible, let your partner know what you want, because he's not a mind reader. All you need now is just a little bit of faith. You'll get through this phase before you know it.

Even though transition is usually the most painful part of labor, some women hardly feel any pain at all. Even so, the contractions will occur more frequently and closer together. The intensity of the contractions also increases. It's almost time to meet your baby!

At this stage, some women respond really well to the touch of their loved one, while others just want to be alone. Let your partner know what you want them to do for you, especially as your desires and needs might change from one moment to the next.

Second Stage of Labor

As you approach the end of transition and the beginning of the second stage of labor, you may feel a powerful sensation to push. In fact, it will probably feel as if you're about to have a bowel movement. If you don't want to catch your baby in the toilet, don't go to the bathroom at this point. This enormous amount of pressure is a significant sign you're getting to the end now. Your baby is moving down the birth canal and ready to be born.

We commonly refer to the second stage of labor as the pushing stage, because you push your baby out. However, pushing is optional and not required to give birth to your baby. Some people recommend laboring down instead of actively pushing, which means letting the contractions take care of birthing the baby.

In a hospital setting or even with a midwife, your provider will probably tell you when to push. But since you have nobody to tell you when you're fully dilated or when it's time to push at home, you can pay attention to what your body is telling you to do. You can breathe through the contractions without pushing, but it may not be possible.

During my first unassisted birth, I wanted to labor down and let my body push the baby out, but the urge to push was much stronger. The pressure was so intense I felt the need to actively push the baby out. With pushing, all you need to remember is to follow your body's lead. Don't push if you don't have the urge to do so, because this may cause your perineum to tear.

Positioning may have something to do with the urge to push. It's a lot easier to ease the baby out when you're giving birth on your hands and knees. This is what I did during my second unassisted birth. While I still felt an urge to push, it was much easier to slow down and just breathe through the contraction.

During labor, your baby will move "two steps forward, one step back."[5] The reason for this is to help you stretch gradually and prevent you from getting tears in your perineum. If you push too hard, you may end up hurting yourself more than necessary. Go with the flow and listen to your body.

When it's time to give birth, choose a suitable position, such as squatting, standing, or being on all fours. If all women were left to follow their natural instincts during labor, only a tiny percentage would choose to labor and give birth while lying on their back. Lying on your back is just not conducive to giving birth, because you have to work against gravity.

During the pushing stage, you should **never**:

- Hold your breath
- Lay on your back
- Push without the urge to do so
- Tug on the umbilical cord

After your baby has moved down the birth canal, you can see and feel him crowning. You can touch your baby's head with your hands, and you can even have someone hand you a mirror to watch the grand entrance. Feeling your baby as he makes his way through is a marvelous sensation. If you remember, you can apply counter pressure on your perineum to help prevent or at least reduce tearing. Your partner can do this for you by using a warm compress.

Many women feel an intense burning sensation when the baby is crowning. They even refer to it as the ring of fire. From the research I've done on this topic, this is a sign from your body to tell you to rest. While you may still have this incredible urge to push, the burning sensation means your tissues are stretching too much.

Not pushing at this point can be incredibly difficult, but taking a break might reduce tearing. Some women never experience this ring of fire, and for the ones who do, it goes away within 30 seconds.

The ring of fire may be the most painful part for you, but now you're almost there. Your baby is being born at this very moment!

After your baby's head is out, it will turn slightly to the side. This makes your baby's shoulders move into position to be born along with the rest of your baby's body. You should probably plan who will catch the baby beforehand. You can do it yourself, or your partner can. If you're close to the floor, such as on your knees, your baby can just slide onto the ground. Make sure the floor is adequately cushioned, just in case.

Once your baby is born, a rush of emotions may overcome you. With the last push, the pain you've experienced will vanish. This allows you to go from moaning and screaming to cooing over your newborn within seconds. Your partner may be amazed at the change, but it's completely natural. You'll feel an intense high, which is difficult to describe. You'll walk on clouds for weeks. The memory of the birth will make you bubble over with joy.

Once your baby has been born, you can take your time to get to know him. If you didn't catch him, you can pick him up and hold him close to you. This is not the time to get dressed. You really need to experience the wonderful warmth of his little body next to yours. It's not just good for the baby.

And as you're cuddling your baby, take time to observe him. Most babies start breathing on their own after they're born, and often they will cry first. This is a good sign, because it clears out their lungs. You can gently wipe any mucus off your baby's face to help him. If your baby was born with the amniotic sac still intact, then you have to rupture it for your baby to breathe.

Keep your baby close to your body and use warm towels or blankets to cover him. If your baby isn't breathing or crying, stroke his back to encourage his systems to work.

Most pregnancies take at least nine months. Labor lasts for several hours, sometimes days. If you include pre-labor contractions, it may feel like you're in labor for several weeks, on and off. In comparison, the event of birth itself is awfully short. The pushing stage can last anywhere from a few minutes to several hours. It will probably be shorter for second and subsequent births. But even though the birth is over quickly, you're probably going to remember it for many years to come. That's only one reason it's so important to give birth the way you want to.

Don't Suction Your Baby's Mouth and Nose

According to the National Institute for Health and Care Excellence (U.K.), there should be no suction before the baby is born (instead of suctioning as soon as the head emerges). If the infant is in good condition with an AGPAR score of 5 or higher, then there should be no suction after birth.[6]

Previously, the recommendation was to suction all newborns after the head was born, but this is no longer recommended according to the American Congress of Obstetricians and Gynecologists. In fact, if the newborn is healthy and vigorous, suctioning can be harmful.[7]

Suction bulbs are commonly used at births in the United States, whether the birth takes place in a hospital or at home. However, current research states the use of suction bulbs is contraindicated. According to The Society of Obstetricians and Gynaecologists of Canada, suctioning causes the baby to gasp or inhale deeply[8], which is clearly not the intention of administering physicians and midwives. Suctioning may interfere with the initiation of breastfeeding, cause tissue trauma, and lower the baby's heart rate.[9]

If you hadn't considered this before, it maybe come as a surprise to you that suctioning a baby is a rough invasion.[10] The mouth of a newborn baby is extremely sensitive. In fact, it's the body part the infant has the most control over. Not only is the mouth used to satisfy hunger and thirst, but it's also how the infant communicates with you. You don't need to conduct a study or hold a degree to understand why using a suction bulb would feel unpleasant or worse to a newborn baby. In most cases, suctioning a newborn isn't just unnecessary, but it can even be harmful to your baby. Of course, if the baby is having trouble breathing, suctioning may be necessary.

How to Examine Your Newborn at Birth

Doctors and midwives usually assign an Apgar score to newborn babies one and five minutes after birth. The Apgar score measures heart rate, respiratory effort, muscle tone, reflexes, and color of the newborn baby. Each area is scored with 0, 1, or 2 points. The total number of points is 10, and most healthy newborns score between 8 and 10. When you examine your baby after an unassisted birth at home, you don't have to assign a score. The scoring system is just a way to quickly determine if a newborn needs medical attention. But it's not a bad idea to pay attention to these five areas.

Respiratory Effort

You can easily examine the respiratory effort of your baby while you're holding him. In fact, this is one of the first signs you're looking for after birth. Obviously, your baby needs to breathe. While not all newborn babies cry, a crying baby is breathing. But your baby may just lie there quietly without having difficulties breathing. Here, you can observe the movement of your baby's chest. If your baby is not breathing at all, you must act fast, because humans cannot survive long without oxygen. Your baby should breathe on his own within the first minute of being born.

Color

Make sure your baby is not limp, grey, or dark in color. Otherwise, he's not getting enough oxygen. This means you'll probably observe poor respiratory effort. If your baby's hands and feet are still grey or blue, that's okay as long as his body is getting color. However, it shouldn't take long for hands and feet to perk up. Within the first hour of life, as circulation improves, their skin will get rosier or darken (depending on ethnicity).

Heart Rate

Your newborn baby's heart rate should be above 100 beats per minute. You can check the heart rate by finding the pulse on your baby's upper arm or by putting your ear next to your baby's chest. While there's nothing wrong with checking your baby's heart rate, it's probably not as helpful as observing your baby's respiratory effort and color. Detecting and accurately measuring your baby's heart rate might not be rocket science, but for a new parent it's not the easiest thing to do, either. It also takes more time than observing your newborn for other signs and prevents you from reacting quickly when necessary.

Muscle Tone

As you're observing your baby, you'll notice he's actively flexing his arms and legs. This is a sign of good muscle tone and just what you want to observe. If your baby is listless and not moving, it's a cause for concern.

Reflexes

Finally, to assign an Apgar score, the doctor or midwife will look for signs of reflexes or irritability. To score well in this area, your baby will offer a good cry, and most babies are happy to comply here. Your baby may not cry at birth, but he'll probably show some reaction to being born, even if it's just a grimace.

What's Important

First, you must ensure your baby is breathing. You can perform a more thorough examination later (where you'll count all the fingers and toes, etc.). Immediately after birth, the priority is to ensure your baby's getting enough oxygen. The best indicators are seeing the baby breathe (or cry) and watching his skin color perk up.

If your baby is not recovering quickly, you need to take action. Before you give birth, educate yourself about newborn CPR and mouth-to-mouth, so you know what to do. Your baby should breathe within the first minute of being born. This is known as the Golden Minute. Otherwise, he needs to be supplied with oxygen before that first minute is over. This is crucial to his survival. I don't want to scare you, but you need to know this, so you can act quickly.

When to Transfer to the Hospital

With giving birth, there are no guarantees. That's true for most of life. But since you've taken charge of your own birth, you need to know when you could really use a helping hand. You can transfer to the hospital anytime you want, but definitely get medical attention if any of the following applies to you and/or your baby:

- Fever
- Blood loss prior to birth
- If baby's heart rate is too low or too high
- Postpartum hemorrhage
- Pale/grey skin or grey lips
- Retained placenta
- Newborn who can't maintain temperature
- Newborn anomalies

Third Stage of Labor

Now that your baby is born, you have time to bond with her. If your baby is willing, you can nurse her. Breastfeeding helps your uterus contract, which will help you enter the last stage of labor and birth the placenta. Pushing the placenta out will not be painful at all, because it's squishy and much smaller than your baby.

There's one important rule you need to obey with birthing the placenta: never pull on the umbilical cord. There's no rush for the placenta to be born. Too often, doctors and midwives alike hurry this process along. At the hospital, they often expect the placenta within minutes of giving birth. However, in a different setting, it may take a lot longer.

According to Sarah Buckley, there are many disadvantages to interfering with the third stage of labor. For best results, all women should have a natural third stage, which includes delaying cord clamping (or omitting it altogether) and allowing the mother to birth her own placenta when she's ready. The mother and baby should be left alone and given time to bond peacefully after birth.[11]

The appearance of the placenta can take quite some time. For the first hour, you have nothing to worry about, unless you're losing a lot of blood or feel faint. If it has been over an hour, and you haven't birthed the placenta, you can try a few things to help it along. First, nursing your baby will encourage contractions. Next, get on all fours or squat. Sometimes, the placenta is just sitting in the vagina's opening and changing positions could be all that's needed for it to make an appearance. And if nothing else works, you can massage your uterus to encourage it to contract.

Once your placenta has been born, examine it for tears. It should be all in one piece. There are three twists in the placenta you can try to locate, two arteries and one vein. The placenta should be complete, because retained placenta in your uterus is not a good thing.

After you've finished examining the placenta, you can keep it (for example, to eat it or encapsulate it), or bury it in your garden. And now it's time to take a deep breath. You just gave birth. Even though lots of people do it, only few women do so unassisted. It's time to rest and get to know your new family member. And of course, you can get up and go to the bathroom and take a shower whenever you want to. In the meantime, your partner can cuddle your newborn baby.

Umbilical Care

After you birth the placenta, you can cut the cord if you haven't done so already. Wait until it stops pulsating and becomes limp and pale. And while the exact moment when you cut the cord is up to you, please don't cut it right away, because it's still your baby's life support. By now, even most hospitals have realized the importance of the umbilical cord, and they offer at least somewhat delayed cord clamping.

If you wait long enough, you won't have to tie off the cord. Once it's pale and limp, there won't be much blood. Otherwise, tie off the cord with shoestring within six inches of your baby's belly. Then you tie it off again, another inch or two from there. Use sterilized scissors to cut in the middle. Later, after your baby has nursed, whenever you're ready to weigh him, you can use an umbilical cord clamp to shorten the umbilical cord attached to his belly. Instead of a clamp, you can use an umbilical cord ring, dental tape, or string.

You don't have to cut the cord if you don't want to. With a lotus birth, you don't cut the cord at all. The placenta stays attached until the cord falls off on its own (usually within the same time frame the stump would fall off). While it can be inconvenient to have the cord with placenta attached to your baby, having a lotus birth encourages you to rest with your baby. A lotus birth is also about respecting the bond between the baby and the placenta and allowing for a peaceful transition for the baby. The downside is limited mobility and having to take the placenta wherever the baby goes.

While you certainly don't have to have a lotus birth, there's absolutely no rush to cut the cord. The longer you wait, the better it will be for your baby. If you're interested in having a Lotus birth, I would encourage you to check out the following website for more details: http://www.mothercultureone.com/lotus-birth.html.

Most sources recommend using salt or certain herbs or both to preserve the placenta and prevent unpleasant smells. Keep the placenta in a bowl or wrap it in a piece of breathable cloth.

The Breast Crawl

Newborns have amazing abilities. Did you know most healthy newborns can find their mother's nipple, latch on, and suckle all on their own if placed on their mother's abdomen after birth? This phenomenon is called the newborn breast crawl. It's a peaceful way to transition from the womb to life with you, because it allows your baby to determine when he's ready to nurse.

For your baby to perform the breast crawl, he needs to rest on your belly while you are in a reclined position. This gives the two of you an excellent chance to bond and cuddle. To promote the breast crawl, keep visitors away, at least during the first hour or until breastfeeding has been established.

Caring for Yourself after Birth

You just gave birth, and your emotions are running high. Lots of hormones are surging through your body, and you should be proud of yourself. You've just accomplished a miracle. This euphoria after giving birth is the climax you deserve after your long pregnancy. You might float on a cloud for several weeks to a few months. Savor the time with your baby while you can and put other projects on the back burner.

You must take care of yourself, now more than ever. There will be contractions after the birth—now called afterpains—which feel like menstrual cramps. The afterpains are caused by your uterus shrinking and expelling its contents at the same time. Your uterus, felt right below your navel, should feel hard. If not, try massaging it.

Afterpains can be quite painful and last for several days after giving birth. A heating pad may bring temporary relief. If it doesn't help, you can take over-the-counter Ibuprofen or Tylenol. It's not unusual for afterpains to be worse after the second or subsequent baby is born. The uterus is working hard, because it has a lot of shrinking to do. Rest as much as possible and focus on your newborn to take your mind off the pain. Empty your bladder frequently to help the uterus contract more efficiently.[12] You may find the intensity of your cramps increasing during your nursing sessions. This is perfectly normal and has to do with the production of oxytocin during breastfeeding.

Giving birth doesn't sound too daunting, does it? Having a baby is something your body already knows how to do, even though you may have never done it before. As long as you treat birth as a natural and maybe even slightly magical event, you'll do just fine.

During all four of my natural births, I was in pain right until the baby was born. But immediately after giving birth, I felt wonderful and was ready to repeat the experience. That's how powerful hormones can be. For some women, it may take a little longer than two seconds after giving birth for wanting to do it again. But most women can have their babies naturally.

To ensure you and your newborn are in good health, you can schedule an appointment with your family doctor within the next couple of days. A family doctor or a pediatrician can listen to your baby's heart and lungs and verify he's healthy. If you have questions about your baby's umbilical cord, soft spots on his head, rashes, acne, or anything else, a good doctor should be able to put your mind at ease.

If you want to get a tear in your perineum stitched, it has to be done within 24 hours of giving birth. However, for a small tear, it may be best to leave it alone and let it heal on its own. There will be more information about vaginal tearing in an upcoming chapter.

Another thing a doctor can do for you during a vaginal exam after birth is to ensure your uterus is shrinking the way it should. You don't need to have this exam done if you don't want to. It's not pleasant, and it's usually unnecessary. If you see a doctor after an unassisted birth, you also risk being offered additional invasive procedures. This is because the doctor could not evaluate your placenta, and therefore, he can't be sure whether you retained any of it.

With traditional medical care, you would normally have another postpartum check-up about six weeks after giving birth. By then, you should no longer be bleeding and any tears will have healed. This check-up usually includes a vaginal exam, and the doctor will probably offer you a prescription for birth control if you so desire. Again, it's up to you whether you want to schedule this check-up or not.

Newborn Evaluation

Newborns will be examined thoroughly within 24 hours of being born if you give birth with a doctor or a midwife. Getting your baby checked out is not a bad idea. A thorough examination should reveal any medical concerns your baby might have, allowing you to take appropriate action if necessary. But how do you perform a newborn exam? I'll take you through the process, step by step. The goal is to examine your newborn thoroughly, looking for symmetry along the way and noticing any deviation from the norm (which isn't always a cause for concern).

Taking Measurements

During a newborn exam, your baby's measurements are taken first. You should weigh your baby naked for accuracy. To do this, you'll have to purchase an infant scale ahead of time. The scale is also useful for tracking weight gain over time, as your baby grows.

To measure your baby's length, I recommend flexible measuring tape (typically used for sewing). You need to measure your baby from the top of her head to the heel of her foot to get accurate results. You may get a slightly different result each time you measure, because newborns curl up. Straighten her out as best as you can or measure your baby's length in segments.

To figure out your baby's head circumference, you'll have to measure the widest area of the head. There's no rush to get this done. It's more important to bond with your baby than to measure her. But don't skip the measurements, because you'll probably need them to get a birth certificate later.

Examining Your Baby

Examine your baby when she's naked, but make sure she doesn't get cold when you do this. You can either use a blanket to cover her up as soon as you're done examining each area and/or keep the room nice and warm. You'll be examining your baby's skin, arms and legs, head and face, and genitals. Doctors will usually inspect the abdomen and check the size and position of various internal organs, including the kidneys, liver, and spleen.

Your Baby's Skin

Your baby's skin should be reddish or dark (depending on ethnicity). However, hands and feet might have a grey or blue tinge to them for the first few hours because of poor blood circulation.[13] Use this opportunity to check for birthmarks or lesions.

Over the next few days, you'll want to watch your baby for signs of jaundice. A baby with jaundice will appear yellow in the face, but the color can move down to the chest, belly, and even to the soles of the feet. Jaundice clears up on its own. Frequent feedings (which are inevitable with newborns) are necessary to keep your baby hydrated. If the soles of your baby's feet turn yellow or the jaundice is severe (very bright yellow) or doesn't clear up after two weeks, then you need to take your baby to the doctor.[14]

Head

Your baby's head may be slightly squashed or molded from his journey through the birth canal. This should resolve within 48 hours.

Gently examine the fontanel, the soft spot on your baby's head. It should be neither sunken nor bulging.

Next, evaluate your baby's face, eyes, and ears. Do you notice any abnormalities of facial form or asymmetry? Are your baby's ears at a normal level, or are they low set (this could be a sign of Down syndrome)?

Doctors will usually perform a red reflex test to detect "vision- and potentially life-threatening abnormalities."[15] This test is performed using an ophthalmoscope, which projects a light onto both eyes at the same time in a darkened room. This is a test you can ask your pediatrician or general practitioner to perform in a few days.

You'll want to evaluate your baby's mouth and check the color of her gums. By now, you probably already know whether your baby's suckling reflex works since your baby will have nursed, but you can gently insert a finger into your baby's mouth to check her palate for abnormalities.

This is also a good time to check for potential tongue or lip ties. A baby with a tongue tie will have trouble breastfeeding long enough, because the tongue can't come out. Not every pediatrician and pediatric dentist knows to look for these. Fortunately, if you treat them right away, you can still salvage your breastfeeding relationship. Otherwise, you may resort to pumping and bottle feeding.

Arms and Legs

Examine your baby's arms, hands, legs, and feet, count fingers and toes, and check for abnormalities. Sometimes, babies are born with additional fingers or toes or fused digits. When you're looking at your baby's hand, count the palmar creases. A single palmar crease may be normal, but it can be a sign for Down syndrome[16]. Check your baby's neck, shoulders, and clavicles for possible birth injuries.

Heart and Lungs

If you have a stethoscope, you can use it to listen to your baby's heart and lungs. Newborn babies have a much higher heart rate than adults. In fact, there's a pretty wide range of what's considered a normal heart rate for newborns. A newborn heart rate can range between 90 and 180, respiratory rate 40-60, and systolic blood pressure 60-90.[17]

Newborn babies sometimes have a heart murmur, because the pattern of circulation changes drastically after birth from life inside the womb. "There are two types of heart murmurs: innocent murmurs and abnormal murmurs. A person with an innocent murmur has a normal heart. This type of heart murmur is common in newborns and children.[...] Innocent heart murmurs may disappear over time, or they may last your entire life without ever causing further health problems."[18]

Abdomen and Back

Experienced practitioners can palpate the abdomen and feel for internal organs. While you might not have the knowledge to do this, you can check your baby's back and abdomen for unusual signs. Again, you're looking for symmetry, especially along the baby's spine. You'll want to examine the umbilical stump over the next few days to check for signs of infection.

A physician would check your baby's hips by utilizing the Ortolani or Barlow maneuver (or both).[19] The hip is a ball and socket joint. The femur (thighbone) may slip out of the socket if the socket is too shallow, which is the case in some infants. Simply put, a doctor will move your baby's thighbones to ensure the hip joint isn't dislocated. If you suspect a problem with his hip joints, please seek medical care for your baby to avoid problems later on.[20]

Genitals

A newborn's genitals may be swollen and dark-colored, because your baby was exposed to your hormones before birth. For the same reason, you may see engorged breasts and white or slightly bloody vaginal discharge in girls.[21] All of this will disappear during the first few weeks.

For boys, you'll want to check the scrotum for undescended testicles. It's important to ensure your baby can eliminate. Verify the opening of the penis is on the top side, but never attempt to pull back your baby boy's foreskin.

For both genders, you want to verify the opening to the anus looks normal. You'll know everything is okay as soon as you have your first wet and poopy diapers.

If you watch your baby boy pee, make sure there's only one stream of urine instead of two. For baby girls, you need to wipe front to back during diaper changes to prevent introducing bacteria into her vagina. Otherwise, your baby's genitals do not require any special care.

Reflexes

It's time to check your baby's reflexes. You can do this by closely observing your baby. It's easy to ensure your baby has sucking, rooting, and grasping reflexes. Another important newborn reflex is the Moro reflex. When your baby experiences the sensation of falling, he will spread out his arms and legs and maybe even cry.[22]

What to Watch For

- Wide separation of fontanels
- Sunken or bulging fontanels
- Third fontanel
- Abnormally shaped or placed ears
- Single palmar crease
- Abnormalities of face, ears, or jaw

Some abnormalities may have a significant underlying cause. For example, a single palmar crease can indicate Down syndrome (although it doesn't have to). You may want to take your baby to a doctor regardless, just to verify everything's okay. Your doctor will listen to your baby's heart and lungs. And if you so desire, you can get a newborn screening done at the same time.

Newborn Screening

If you take your baby to the doctor, they may offer you a newborn screening (PKU). For the screening, your baby's blood will be evaluated for metabolic disorders otherwise not apparent at birth. For this purpose, they'll draw blood from your baby's foot.

A thoughtful pediatrician will warm your baby's foot beforehand. Warming up the area encourages blood to flow to the foot. This means the blood can be drawn quickly. If you decide to have this screening done, you may want your partner to be with your baby and bring her to you afterwards for a comforting nursing session. It's difficult to watch someone poke your baby's foot and cause her to cry.

Other newborn procedures performed at the hospital include the Vitamin K shot and the antibiotic eye ointment. I've already discussed the side effects of both. Personally, I believe healthy babies are born perfect and don't need any routine medical procedures at birth. But if your baby needs medical attention for other reasons, please obtain it right away.

Birthing Cheat Sheet

You can find a printable version of this birthing cheat sheet on my website www.TheUnassistedBaby.com under Resources.

Early Labor To-Do List

- Sterilize scissors, shoestring, etc.
- Put towels in the dryer
- Have a clock or watch ready
- Timer or stopwatch for checking baby's pulse (optional)
- Set up labor area
- Put Peri bottle in the bathroom
- Make the bed

After Birth: Baby Evaluation

- Record date and exact time:
- Is baby breathing / crying?
- Is your baby's skin turning rosy red or darkening (depending on ethnicity)?
- Baby's pulse (optional):

How to check your baby's pulse: Use the baby's brachial artery, which is on the upper arm between the elbow and shoulder. For best accuracy, count for 30 seconds, then multiply result by 2 to get beats per minute. If your baby is too squirmy, count for 15 seconds and multiply by 4.

The baby's pulse can range anywhere from 110 to 160. A pulse below 100 can be concerning.

Umbilical Cord Procedure

Tie off the cord with shoestring within six inches from your baby's navel. Tie it off again another inch or two from there and then use scissors to cut in the middle. Later, after your baby has nursed, when you're ready to weigh him, use the clamp to shorten the umbilical cord attached to his belly.

Placenta Evaluation

- Ensure the placenta is in one piece
- Locate three twists in the placenta (2 arteries and one vein)

Measuring Baby

Length:

Measure your baby from the top of his head to the heel of his foot. Do this in sections since he'll likely squirm. Straighten him out as best as possible for increased accuracy.

Weight:

Weigh baby naked for increased accuracy.

Head Circumference:

Measure the largest area of his head.

Concerns during Labor and Birth

I've already discussed dealing with your fears in an earlier chapter. There are many things for a first-time mother and even a veteran mom to be afraid of. There are a lot of irrational fears (sometimes reflected in weird pregnancy dreams), and there are some legitimate fears. While I may not mention every concern you harbor around birth, it doesn't mean you can't find a solution elsewhere. Do your research and confront your fear by finding an answer.

Imagine the worst-case scenario. What would you do? Is there a way to prevent it from happening? Finally, think about the likelihood of it happening. Is it just a remote possibility in the first place? Then don't worry about it and maybe look at cute baby clothes instead.

Baby Not Breathing

Even though neither of my first two children had breathing problems at birth, I worried about my baby not breathing when I was planning my first unassisted birth. It all began when I heard a sad birth story, which is probably another reason to only listen to positive birth stories.

For my first two births, I had relied on a doctor and then a midwife to handle any complications. It never even crossed my mind something might go wrong, although the presence of a birth attendant doesn't prevent problems.

Thankfully, I have an extremely supportive husband who loves finding solutions. Midwives and hospitals use oxygen devices for the baby until they can get her to breathe on her own. What if this device wasn't there? The solution is simple: CPR. My husband had been CPR-certified in the past, and he's also a great person to have around in an emergency. We decided for him to take a CPR course to freshen up his skills, and this time, he would focus on infant CPR. This relieved my fears immensely.

You don't have to be CPR-certified. If you're already familiar with administering CPR, even an online refresher course could be enough. It all depends on what you feel comfortable with. Just remember CPR for infants is not the same as for adults. For example, you cannot use as much pressure on their chest.

Some newborns may need a little help to get going without needing full CPR. A few tricks often work with newborns. You can change their position, so that their head is lower than their body. Sometimes, flicking their feet can help if they don't start breathing right away. Clear your baby's airways by gently wiping away the mucus from her face. You can rub her back to get her systems going. You may need to give a puff of air into the baby's mouth and nose to encourage them to react and breathe on their own, but don't blow hard. Use small puffs of air in one-second intervals. If the baby doesn't respond quickly, you need to start full CPR with chest compressions.

According to the American Academy of Pediatrics, about 10% of babies require some help to breathe at birth, but less than 1% requires extensive resuscitative measures.[23] Within the first minute of life you need to warm the baby, clear his airways if needed, dry the baby, and stimulate him (rubbing his back). If he doesn't start breathing within the first 60 seconds, you need to offer oxygen to the baby. "Rescuers should ensure that assisted ventilation is being delivered optimally before starting chest compressions."[24]

Look into infant CPR to prepare, just in case. If you need to administer CPR, the other person present should call 911. If you had a midwife attending your birth, she would have some sort of oxygen device to use until the ambulance arrived. You can provide the same emergency care, as long as you prepare ahead of time. If you're really concerned, you may even rent such an oxygen tank. Just make sure you know how to use it.

Generally, there's no need to worry overly much. A healthy, full-term baby will start breathing on his own, even if you have to give him a little nudge first.

Breech Baby

There are many birth stories with happy endings involving breech babies. Generally, babies come out head first, but even if they decide to change their position and come out butt first, things usually turn out just fine. Only 3-4% of babies are breech at 40 weeks of gestation.[25]

Unfortunately, a breech baby results in a caesarean section for most women. This is partly because doctors aren't trained to help women give birth to breech babies anymore. Presumably, they opt for C-sections to avoid getting sued. However, C-sections come with their own enormous risks for both mother and baby.

There are unique positions and techniques which may help you turn a baby before birth. The website www.spinningbabies.com is currently the best online resource I have found on this topic. Some babies will turn on their own right before labor. And many babies are born bottom first with no issues at all. If you give birth in a hospital in the traditional position, you may have a hard time with a breech baby. In fact, most doctors may not even let you give birth to a breech baby vaginally and talk you into having a C-section, unless you show up at the hospital ready to push.

Sometimes it's possible to turn a baby manually inside the womb. An experienced midwife may attempt it for you, but it's not clear when to do this. Some sources recommend turning the baby before she is full-term, because it's easier to turn her. Others say the baby will turn right back if you do this before 37 weeks. Then again, some sources recommend not turning a baby until 37 weeks.

If you're unsure about your baby's position, you can schedule a prenatal appointment to check. You can also try to determine the baby's position yourself. In the later stages of pregnancy (when you're closer to your due date), you can lie on your back and feel for the baby. First, focus on where you feel kicks (tiny movements could be hands or feet). You should be able to determine where your baby's back is, because his spine is rather big and hard. For a baby who is head down, you can feel his head right above your pubic bone. Your partner could have an easier time feeling for the baby than you, so let him try it, too.

If you still don't know where your baby's head is, there's something else you can try. You can feel for your baby vaginally. The best place to do this is on the toilet. After washing your hands, you can gently guide your index or middle finger (whichever one will reach better) inside and feel for the vaginal wall. You have to reach pretty high up inside of you, until you feel something round and hard. If your baby is head down, you may feel the ridges on his head. One ridge goes from the front to the back of the head. Even if you're unsure whether you felt his head or his butt, feeling something hard means your baby is not transverse (horizontally) breech. A baby that lies horizontally is in the only position you cannot give birth to naturally.

The most important thing to know about giving birth to a breech baby:

- Get into a favorable position such as standing, squatting, or on all fours.
- Don't let anyone touch you or the baby during birth. This can disrupt the process and cause a lot of harm.[26]
- Above all, have faith! Your baby knows what he's doing.

While giving birth to a breech baby, you must never have unsupportive staff around you. Using forceps or trying to extract the baby may hurt his spine or head, since the head is born last.

"During a vaginal birth, having the head come out last increases the risk that the umbilical cord will be compressed or prolapsed. A compressed cord is not able to provide oxygen to the baby. Additionally, because the head is coming out neck first, it is less likely to mold increasing the risk for the head to get stuck."[27]

According to Henci Goer[28], birthing a breech baby vaginally is a reasonable choice, because poor outcomes for breech babies have nothing to do with the birth route. They may be breech because of a health condition, but the choice of birth doesn't really help their condition. On the contrary, C-sections don't remove the risks of a breech birth, and they increase maternal risk unnecessarily. To have a successful breech birth, Henci Goer advises women to hire a skilled, gentle birth attendant, monitor the fetal heart rate closely, and to delay pushing until full dilation. The latter ensures your baby will fit through the birth canal without getting stuck on the way.

The biggest takeaway for breech births: "For a normal breech birth the time-honoured advice, **hands off the breech**, is still the safest advice."[29]

Umbilical Cord Prolapse

If the umbilical cord comes out before your baby, you need to have an emergency C-section. Otherwise, your baby will not get enough oxygen as the cord is compressed during the contractions.

If you have an urge to push when the umbilical cord falls out of the vagina alone, bear down as hard and as quickly as possible. If there's no urge to push, get on your knees with your chest to the floor to relieve pressure on the chord. The chord can be loosely wrapped in a warm, moist towel. In this position, you need to be taken to the hospital right away for an immediate C-section[30].

One cause for umbilical cord prolapse is the premature rupture of the membranes. Other potential causes include a breech birth, a birth involving multiples, an excessive amount of amniotic fluid, or an abnormally long umbilical cord.

Tearing

Tearing was one of my fears I had to conquer before I could give birth unassisted. I had perineal tears with both of my daughters, even though my first baby only weighed 4 pounds. I was afraid of tearing, because I really wanted to avoid medical interventions. For both of my previous births, I had received stitches, but I really wanted to have this baby at home on my own. I didn't want to go to the hospital immediately after the birth for stitches.

I ended up reading a lot about tears in the perineum prior to my first unassisted birth. Here are the most common suggestions for preventing tears:

- Perineal massage before birth
- Laboring down
- Hands-and-knees position for birth
- Perineal support during birth
- Paying attention to your body and your baby

Some providers recommend performing perineal massages daily, starting at about six weeks before your due date. This is supposed to help stretch the tissues. The basic idea is to massage and stretch your vagina and perineum using olive oil, almond oil, K-Y jelly, Vitamin E oil, or wheat germ oil. When it's time to give birth, your perineum is less likely to tear.[31]

After giving instructions for doing perineal massage, prenatal massage therapist Tiffany Alblinger says: "Notice I omitted the 'apply pressure until you feel a burning sensation to ensure you are getting a good stretch' as this may possibly be creating microtears and damaging the tissue."[32] Most instructions recommend doing it until you feel the burning sensation, which is precisely the point when you might cause damage to your perineum.

Whether you believe perineal massage to be helpful to prevent tearing isn't the only deciding factor. In fact, most women absolutely hate performing perineal massage. It's an unnatural thing to do, and it doesn't feel good. Fortunately, there are other options available to you.

For many women, perineal support during labor helps prevent tearing. During labor, you can use a warm compress on your perineum, while providing some counter-pressure during pushing. You can make a compress the following way: Use an old washcloth or a piece of flannel and put it in cold-pressed castor oil. Next, you wring out the cloth and put it on your perineum, then cover it up with something waterproof. You can put a heating pad on top of it if you like. Alternatively, you can use a warm washcloth and press it against your perineum as you're giving birth.[33] Either way, when using counter-pressure, you're not trying to push the baby back in. Instead, you're helping your perineum stay intact by letting it stretch slowly.

A good birthing position can prevent tearing. Lying on your back will not prevent tears. Instead, give birth on all fours. According to Rachel Reed, independent midwife, "lateral and hands-knees positions reduce the chance of tearing and supine, squatting or lithotomy positions increase the chance of tearing."[34] Apparently, many women will instinctively move to a hands and knees position if left alone just before the head is crowning.

With my second unassisted birth, I ended up in the hands-knees position, too. I reminded myself not to push as the head was crowning, and in that position, it wasn't difficult. While nobody examined me afterwards, this was the least pain I ever experienced after having a baby. This leads me to believe I had only minimal tearing or none.

Being aware of your baby's progress may be the most important part. If you're pushing when someone else tells you to, and neither looking at nor touching your vagina, you won't know how flexible you are. In fact, some midwives ask their pregnant clients, long before it's time to give birth, to assess the tightness of their perineum in different positions and find out when it's most flexible. This lets them figure out for themselves what a good birthing position might be.

Remember, you're allowed to touch your perineum during labor and birth. It's your body. When you use your hands to feel, you can experience how much your skin is stretching. And you can apply some counter pressure and feel your baby's head for the first time. It's such an amazing feeling to touch your baby as he's born.

While you're birthing your baby, it helps to take a deep breath sometimes. It might be easier to opt for just one more big push to get it over with and disregard the consequences of vaginal tears. But if you take it slow instead, breathe through the contractions, and let your uterus take care of the pushing, you'll have a better chance of an intact perineum.

Now what happens if you still end up with a tear? It turns out tears can range from first to fourth degree in severity. A first-degree tear is very minor, while a fourth-degree tear goes all the way down to your rectum. A fourth-degree tear is something you would want to get treated. However, a fourth-degree tear is highly unlikely if you're giving birth naturally. For a tear involving your rectum, you need to go to the hospital and get stitches. If a third or fourth-degree tear is not treated, you may have serious problems with bowel movements later on.

You'll probably need a little mirror to check out the damage (if there is any). And just so you know, the worst perineal tears happen when an episiotomy is performed or when forceps are used.

For a minor first-degree tear, nothing needs to be done. Even a second-degree tear doesn't have to be stitched. Skin injuries can heal on their own. The stitches are only there to keep the skin together, since most people cannot rest for two weeks without running around and doing things. If you end up with a small tear, it's even more important for you to rest in bed with your newborn and let your body heal itself. You may use liquid band-aids for such a tear, but the easiest option is to simply leave it alone.

If you want to get stitches, you can. You'll need to go to the hospital within a few hours after birth. If it has been over 24 hours, the doctor won't stitch your tear because the risk of infection is too great. For stitching a tear, a doctor or midwife will numb the area as best as possible—you'll most likely still feel pain for part of the procedure, because it's tricky to numb the perineum in its entirety.

When you leave a second-degree tear alone to heal, there's a small possibility you might need reconstructive surgery later.[35] You should also know not all midwives are trained to suture perineal tears. In fact, this is one area where OB/GYNs usually have greater skills and experience than midwives. On the other hand, midwives are often better able to help you prevent tears in the first place.

In short, birthing in the hands-and-knees position and leaving minor tears alone are probably your best options. After I learned about perineal tears, I wasn't worried anymore. I ended up with a second-degree tear for my first unassisted birth, but it healed fine on its own. With my second unassisted birth, I don't think I tore at all. My last birth had minor tearing, based on the pain level I experienced. The hands-knees position made all the difference for me. When I assumed a more upright position, I always tore a little, but not badly enough to warrant stitches or other treatment.

Hemorrhage

Excessive blood loss after childbirth is called postpartum hemorrhage. We define excessive blood loss as over 500 ml or 2 cups for a vaginal birth.[36] Hemorrhages are more likely if:

- You have a C-section.
- You've been given Pitocin.
- You have a large baby or multiple babies.
- You've been given anesthesia.

- You've had many children (over 5 term pregnancies).
- The umbilical cord or placenta is pulled on.

I found many sources advising the use of oxytocin as a preventive measure against postpartum hemorrhage. However, artificial oxytocin "can have serious side effects including seizures and heart rhythm irregularities."[37] Even if those side effects are rare, it doesn't sound like a good 'preventive' measure to give to all women in labor, but this is what some hospitals are doing.

The best prevention for postpartum hemorrhage is being in excellent health. Other preventive measures include:

- Don't push until you're fully dilated (listen to your body)
- Stay upright and mobile to shorten labor and birth
- Empty your bladder frequently during labor and afterwards
- Get enough iron in your diet to prevent anemia
- Avoid induction and augmentation of labor and avoid episiotomies[38]
- Never tug on the umbilical cord

The last part deserves special mention. **Don't pull on the umbilical cord.** Doing so could cause your placenta to rupture, which is dangerous to you.

While you always have the option of calling 911 in case of postpartum hemorrhage, there are some herbal remedies to treat hemorrhaging, such as Shepherd's purse. Chewing on a piece of your placenta can also slow the bleeding.

There are a variety of homeopathic treatments for postpartum hemorrhage. I suggest you do your own research and decide what you want to do. You can order some herbal remedies to have on hand afterwards. However, you need to know what to take, how to take it, and what dosage you need.

With extreme blood loss, you need to see immediate results. Otherwise, you really need to call for help.

If you hemorrhage in a hospital setting, the typical treatment is to massage your uterus first and administer oxytocin if needed. The doctor or nurse may attempt to retrieve any remaining pieces of your placenta by inserting their hand into your uterus. According to a friend of mine, this hurts a lot more than giving birth. This is not surprising, considering your cervix is closing and your uterus is already shrinking. If the bleeding can't be stopped, the doctor will perform surgery. And if all else fails, you'll have a hysterectomy (which is the removal of your uterus), preventing you from having any more children.

Don't let the potential dangers of a hemorrhage scare you. Hemorrhages are not common at all (only 5% of women experience them). If you've given birth before without hemorrhaging, there's no reason you can't do it again. If you want to be prepared, have some Shepherd's purse, Bellis perennis (bellis) or Arnica montana (arnica)[39] on hand. If you hire a midwife to attend the birth, you can choose one who has successfully treated hemorrhages in the past. However, you may still end up in the hospital for a hemorrhage, even if there is a midwife present at your birth.

At the very least, you need to be aware of the signs of a hemorrhage, so you can call for help if it happens. Besides uncontrolled bleeding, a woman experiencing postpartum hemorrhage may have decreased blood pressure and an increased heart rate. She may also go into shock.

According to Gregory J. White's "Emergency Childbirth Manual", controlling the bleeding by putting pressure on the uterus should be done after the placenta has been born. And if you're suffering from shock (you may be pale, sweaty, weak, breathing hard, or very thirsty), your partner should keep you cool and with your feet up until the paramedics arrive.[40]

Premature Labor

Premature labor is defined as labor before 37 weeks, but after 20 weeks. If you're having severe cramps long before your due date that don't subside, seek medical attention. According to Trina Pagano, M.D., the risk factors for premature labor include:

- Smoking
- Being extremely overweight or underweight before pregnancy
- Drinking alcohol or using drugs
- Having certain health conditions, such as high blood pressure or diabetes
- Being pregnant with a baby who has certain birth defects
- Being pregnant through in-vitro fertilization
- Having twins or multiples
- Family or personal history of premature labor
- Getting pregnant too soon after having a baby[41]

Your risk of premature labor goes up tremendously if you're unhealthy. But besides taking care of yourself, there's nothing much you can do to prevent either a miscarriage or premature labor.

If you're having contractions before 36 or 37 weeks, you may need to seek help. While you can probably give birth on your own, your baby may not survive at this point without life support. It means your baby's best chance is to be born at the hospital. If you're indeed in labor, you may be given medication intravenously to stop the contractions. They may put you on bed rest. If labor can't be stopped, the hospital staff will try their best to help your baby after he is born.

Try not to worry too much about a miscarriage or premature labor. Instead, focus on is prevention by eating healthy diet. Your body will take care of the rest for you.

When You Need Medical Attention

During Pregnancy

If you're healthy, your pregnancy and birth will most likely go over without a hitch. However, you can seek medical care during your pregnancy whenever you want to. Here are some reasons to see a doctor during your pregnancy:

- If you're taking prescription medications
- If you have a diagnosable disease
- To have some prenatal testing done
- To find out if you're a suitable candidate for a homebirth
- To receive prenatal care
- To find out the baby's position
- If you suspect fetal distress

Even when you seek medical care, you're still the one in charge of your pregnancy. If you only want to have one prenatal visit, that's fine. If you want all of them or none, that's totally okay, too. You need to do whatever you feel most comfortable with.

Midwives evaluate their patients to see if they qualify for a homebirth. But there are a lot of women who want to give birth at home, even if the midwife doesn't consider it safe for them to do so.

Ultimately, you know what your body is capable of better than anyone else. There are many women with successful vaginal births after C-section who accomplished this against medical advice. This doesn't mean you should ignore any and all medical advice. Instead, make educated decisions while taking other people's knowledge and expertise into account.

During Labor and Birth

Even if you didn't have any prenatal care during your pregnancy, there may be a good reason to seek medical attention during labor or even after birth, such as

- Sharp pains which are not labor contractions
- Excessive blood loss of the mother
- Umbilical cord prolapse
- Fever
- Postpartum hemorrhage
- Retained placenta
- Newborn who can't maintain temperature
- Newborn anomalies

A good rule is this: **when in doubt, call for help**. It's better to have medical personnel available than to risk the life of either the mother or the baby. But putting 911 on speed-dial in your phone is not the only preparation you need. If you're not willing to learn about childbirth, then giving birth unassisted is not a good choice for you or your baby.

To have a successful, unassisted birth at home, you need to get ready ahead of time. It's perfectly natural to panic occasionally and maybe even question your sanity. But overall, you should feel comfortable with the idea of birthing at home. If you live in a state of constant fear after deciding to give birth unassisted, you may not be ready to do this on your own yet. You can still give birth at home with a supportive midwife, or you can decide to give birth at the hospital. With proper planning and careful selection of your birth attendant, you can have the peaceful, natural birth you want, even if it's not an unassisted birth.

---

[1] GMA Network (2013). "Some women orgasm during childbirth, study shows." Retrieved from
http://www.gmanetwork.com/news/story/312649/scitech/science/some-women-orgasm-during-childbirth-study-shows.

[2] Brennan, Matthew, MD (2012). "Water Birth: Benefits & Risks." Retrieved from http://www.webmd.com/baby/guide/water-birth?page=1.

[3] BabyCenter L.L.C. (2011). "The stages of labor" Retrieved from http://www.babycenter.com/stages-of-labor?showAll=true.

[4] BabyCenter L.L.C. (2011). "The stages of labor" Retrieved from http://www.babycenter.com/stages-of-labor?showAll=true.

[5] BabyCenter L.L.C. (2011). "The stages of labor" Retrieved from http://www.babycenter.com/stages-of-labor?showAll=true.

[6] National Institute for Health and Care Excellence (2014). Intrapartum care: Care of healthy women and their babies during childbirth. Retrieved from https://www.nice.org.uk/guidance/cg55/chapter/1-guidance#meconium-stained-liquor.

[7] 2005 American Heart Association (AHA) guidelines for cardiopulmonary resuscitation (CPR) and emergency cardiovascular care (ECC) of pediatric and neonatal patients: pediatric basic life support. American Heart Association. Pediatrics 2006;117:e989–1004. http://www.acog.org/Resources-And-Publications/Committee-Opinions/Committee-on-Obstetric-Practice/Management-of-Delivery-of-a-Newborn-With-Meconium-Stained-Amniotic-Fluid

[8] The Society of Obstetricians and Gynecologists of Canada (2009). "Management of Meconium at Birth". Retrieved from http://sogc.org/guidelines/management-of-meconium-at-birth-technical-update/.

[9] Reed, Rachel (2010). The Curse of Meconium Stained Liquor. Retrieved from http://midwifethinking.com/2010/10/09/the-curse-of-meconium-stained-liquor/.

[10] Oral Aversion in the Breastfed Neonate. Linda Killion Healow, BSN, IBCLC and Rebecca Sliter Hugh, IBCLC from Breastfeeding Abstracts, August 2000, Volume 20, Number 1, pp. 3-4. Retrieved from http://www.llli.org/ba/aug00.html.

[11] Buckley, Sarah, J., M.D. (2005). "Leaving Well Alone: A Natural Approach to the Third Stage of labour." Retrieved from http://sarahbuckley.com/leaving-well-alone-a-natural-approach-to-the-third-stage-of-labour.

[12] BabyCenter (2014). "Postpartum: Cramps (afterpains)." Retrieved from http://www.babycenter.com/0_postpartum-cramps-afterpains_11723.bc.

[13] Lawrence, Ruth, MD. Merck Manuals (2006). Physical Examination of the Newborn. Retrieved from http://www.merckmanuals.com/home/childrens_health_issues/care_of_newborns_and_infants/physical_examination_of_the_newborn.html.

[14] U.S. National Library of Medicine (2013). Newborn Jaundice. Retrieved from http://www.nlm.nih.gov/medlineplus/ency/article/001559.htm.

[15] American Academy of Ophthalmology. (2008) Red Reflex Examination in Neonates, Infants and Children. Retrieved from http://www.aao.org/about/policy/upload/Red-Reflex-Testing-2008.pdf

[16] Fuloria M and Keiter S; The Newborn Examination: Part I. Emergencies and Common Abnormalities Involving the Skin, Head, Neck, Chest, and Respiratory and Cardiovascular Systems.; Am Fam Phys 2002;65:61-8.

[17] Merlin C. Lowe, Jr, MD, FAAP, Dale P. Woolridge, MD, PhD, FAAEM, FAAP, FACEP (2007). The Normal Newborn Exam, or Is It? Emerg Med Clin N Am, 25 (2007) 921–946. Retrieved from http://www.ais.up.ac.za/health/blocks/block9/normal.pdf

[18] Mayo Foundation for Medical Education and Research (2014). Heart Murmurs. Retrieved from http://www.mayoclinic.org/diseases-conditions/heart-murmurs/basics/causes/con-20028706.

[19] Sewell MD, Rosendahl K, Eastwood DM; Developmental dysplasia of the hip. BMJ. 2009 Nov 24;339:b4454. doi: 10.1136/bmj.b4454. Retrieved from http://www.ncbi.nlm.nih.gov/pubmed/19934187?dopt=Abstract.

[20] U.S. National Library of Medicine (2014). Developmental dysplasia of the hip. Retrieved from http://www.nlm.nih.gov/medlineplus/ency/article/000971.htm.

[21] David H. Barad, MD, MS, Merck Manuals (2014). Vaginal Bleeding. Retrieved from http://www.merckmanuals.com/home/womens_health_issues/symptoms_of_gynecologic_disorders/vaginal_bleeding.html.

[22] U.S. National Library of Medicine (2013). Infant reflexes. Retrieved from http://www.nlm.nih.gov/medlineplus/ency/article/003292.htm.

[23] American Academy of Pediatrics (2013). "Neonatal Resuscitation: 2010 American Heart Association Guidelines for Cardiopulmonary Resuscitation and Emergency Cardiovascular Care." Retrieved from http://pediatrics.aappublications.org/content/126/5/e1400.full.

[24] American Academy of Pediatrics (2013). "Neonatal Resuscitation: 2010 American Heart Association Guidelines for Cardiopulmonary Resuscitation and Emergency Cardiovascular Care." Retrieved from http://pediatrics.aappublications.org/content/126/5/e1400.full.

[25] American College of Obstetricians and Gynecologists (2000, reaffirmed 2012). External cephalic version. ACOG Practice Bulletin No. 13. Obstetrics and Gynecology, 95(2): 1–7.

[26] Spinning Babies (2013). "Breech: bottoms up – Vaginal breech birth." Retrieved from http://spinningbabies.com/baby-positions/breech-bottoms-up/339-vaginal-breech-birth?showall=1.

[27] Vanderlaan, Jennifer (2013). "Labor Challenge: Breech Position" Retrieved from http://www.birthingnaturally.net/birth/challenges/breech.html.

[28] "The Thinking Woman's Guide to a Better Birth" by Henci Goer

[29] Mary Cronk, MBE. "Keep Your Hands Off the Breech". AIMS Journal Autumn 1998, Vol 10 No 3

[30] White, Gregory: "Emergency Childbirth: A Manual"

[31] American College of Nurse-Midwives (2005). "Perineal Massage in Pregnancy." Retrieved from http://www.midwife.org/ACNM/files/ccLibraryFiles/Filename/000000000656/Perineal%20Massage%20in%20Pregnancy.pdf.

[32] Alblinger, Tiffany (2103). "Perineal Massage." Retrieved from http://www.naturalbabypros.com/article/552/perineal-massage/.

[33] Aasheim V, Nilsen ABVika, Lukasse M, Reinar LM. Perineal techniques during the second stage of labour for reducing perineal trauma. Cochrane Database of Systematic Reviews 2011, Issue 12. Art. No.: CD006672. DOI: 10.1002/14651858.CD006672.pub2.

[34] Albers, LL, Anderson, D, Cragin, L & al, e 1996, 'Factors related to perineal trauma in childbirth',*Journal of Nurse Midwifery*, vol. 41, pp. 269-76.

[35] NHS Foundation Trust (n.d.) "Repair of Perineal Trauma - 1st and 2nd Degree Tears/Episiotomies." Retrieved from http://www.icid.salisbury.nhs.uk/ClinicalManagement/MaternityNeonatal/Pages/RepairofPerinealTrauma-1stand2ndDegreeTearsEpisiotomies.aspx.

[36] Weiss, Robin Elise, LCCE (2014). "Postpartum Hemorrhage." Retrieved from http://pregnancy.about.com/cs/postpartumrecover/a/pph.htm.

[37] Bastyr Center for Natural Health (2013). "Homeopathy Prevents Postpartum Hemorrhage" retrieved from http://www.bastyrcenter.org/content/view/997/.

[38] PATH (2011). "Postpartum hemorrhage prevention and treatment" Retrieved from http://www.pphprevention.org/pph.php.

[39] Bastyr Center for Natural Health (2013). "Homeopathy Prevents Postpartum Hemorrhage". Retrieved from http://www.bastyrcenter.org/content/view/997/.

[40] White, Gregory J., M.D. (1998). "Emergency Childbirth – A Manual."

[41] Pagano, Trina, M.D. (2012). Premature Labor. Retrieved from http://www.webmd.com/baby/premature-labor?page=1.

Chapter 5

After Childbirth

Postpartum Care for You

Before and after childbirth, your body is going through many changes. During pregnancy, the changes occur gradually. Your body has nine months or more to expand and make room for your baby. Your waist size adjusts during pregnancy, but so do your hormone levels and some of your internal organs. Your lungs, stomach, and bladder have to make room for your growing uterus, affecting you directly with shortness of breath, heartburn, and frequent bathroom visits. Once your baby is born, you may be concerned about:

- Bleeding and cramping
- Engorged breasts
- Perineal tenderness
- Your weight and your body image
- Sweating
- Hair Loss
- Incontinence and/or Constipation
- Hemorrhoids
- Feeling blue

I'd love to tell you everything will go back to normal once your baby is born, but it would be a lie. The reality is your body may never be quite the same, although many of the changes are only temporary.

Bleeding and Cramping

After giving birth, you can expect to bleed (much like having your period) for several weeks. This postpartum bleeding is called lochia.

It's basically spring-cleaning for your uterus. After a few days, you'll pass blood clots, too.

Lochia can last anywhere from two to three weeks up to six weeks. Use menstrual pads during this time (no tampons allowed right after childbirth). Your bleeding should get lighter as time goes by. If you engage in strenuous activity, you may find an increase in lochia. This is a sign for you to take it easy. Your body is still in recovery, remember?

If you're bleeding heavily and soaking through more than one pad in an hour or passing blood clots bigger than a golf ball, you need to seek medical attention.[1] Although it's rare, this may be a sign of postpartum hemorrhage.

Lochia only differs from your normal period in its duration. You can think of it as making up for lost time, since you didn't have a regular period during your pregnancy. You can stock up on pads ahead of time to prepare for it. Avoid strenuous exercise for the first six weeks after having your baby and listen to your body's needs for rest and sleep. It's recommended you refrain from having sexual intercourse to give your cervix enough time to close up again properly.

Along with the bleeding, you may experience cramping. This can be quite severe in the first few days after giving birth, and it's all because your uterus is shrinking down to its original size (from about 1000g to 50-100g[2]). It may be especially painful during nursing sessions, because breastfeeding sends those signals to your uterus to contract. Afterpains are often worse with second and subsequent births. For pain relief, try a heating pad and/or take some Ibuprofen or alternative pain medicine.

Even if you normally avoid taking Ibuprofen, you'll probably find afterpains are too painful without any sort of pain reliever. Don't exceed the recommended dosage on the bottle and seek care if it doesn't get better soon. Afterpains usually subside within a few days of giving birth.

Engorged Breasts

Bigger breasts may be one change in your body you (and your partner) appreciate. Because of the production of breastmilk, your breasts will become engorged about two to three days after your baby is born. They may become painful to the touch. An ice pack can bring relief, but your milk production will adjust by itself in time. Until then, you'll need extra nursing pads.

To avoid leaking breastmilk through your clothes, try the following: Before you nurse your baby, replace the wet nursing pads on the side your baby is not feeding on. While your baby is nursing on one side, the other breast will leak milk, too. But if you put in a fresh nursing pad before the nursing session, it may soak up the extra milk. Otherwise, you'll end up with some wet spots on your shirt. Fortunately, breastmilk washes right out and doesn't stain, but wet spots can still be embarrassing and annoying, especially in public. There are also special cups you can buy instead of nursing pads, which allow you to collect the breastmilk and store it for later.

With the production of breastmilk, your appetite and thirst will increase. Now you'll finally have room to eat a big meal. You'll probably be hungry at all hours. This is perfectly normal since you're feeding your little one around the clock. As long as you drink plenty of water and satisfy your hunger with healthy snacks and meals throughout the day, you can eat whenever you feel hungry. Have some midnight snacks handy as well, especially during the first few weeks. When you're frequently up throughout the night, it's not realistic to forego food until the morning. This isn't promoting gluttony, because it's about temporarily adjusting to what your body needs to make it through these first few hard weeks with a newborn.

Perineal Tenderness

Even if you didn't tear or had only minor tearing, your perineum will probably be tender for a while after giving birth. This may make you feel reluctant to use the bathroom. It might even sting when you urinate. To relieve any painful sensations, use a squirt bottle and squirt warm water on your perineum while you're urinating. It sounds weird, but it really works. And the stinging pain will go away after a couple of days. Until then, you can use that squirt bottle, but please go to the bathroom when you need to instead of holding it in.

Another big milestone is your first bowel movement after you give birth. It may not happen the day you give birth, but a day or two afterwards. Eating foods high in fiber and drinking plenty of water will ensure you don't get constipated. For the first bowel movement, it's recommended not to strain too hard or at all. Otherwise, it could be painful, especially if you have any perineal tears (whether or not you had stitches).

Your Weight and Body Image

You probably won't be back to your pre-pregnancy weight immediately after giving birth. However, you can expect to lose about 10 to 15 pounds all at once. This weight includes the weight of your baby, the placenta, and some other bodily fluids you're shedding. It will probably take longer than six weeks to get rid of all those pregnancy pounds, but don't get discouraged. It took nine months to gain it, and it may take the same amount of time or longer to get rid of it.

Weight loss will differ for every woman. Breastfeeding may help since you're burning tons of extra calories, but it can also make you hungrier. As long as you're eating a healthy diet, don't worry too much about your weight, especially in the first few weeks after giving birth. After going through pregnancy and childbirth, your body is going to look different. Many women still look pregnant after giving birth. It takes time for the uterus to shrink, and this can contribute to making your belly look bloated.

After the first six weeks, you can start an exercise routine again and set reasonable weight loss goals for yourself. Unfortunately, some things don't go away with exercise and diet. For example, you may never have a perfect bikini body again due to stretch marks and extra belly fat.

Although I don't suggest you get hung up over the changes in your body, I'm not advocating you just "let yourself go". It will make you feel better if you get a nice top and pair of pants that fit you now, because you most likely won't fit into your pre-pregnancy size just yet. Having at least one nice outfit will make you feel more attractive, and therefore, happier. Otherwise, focus on eating healthy without counting calories. Once you're able to, get active. Having a baby is a good excuse to walk in the park, no matter what the weather is like. Your baby will sleep much better if you're on the move, either in the stroller or in a sling. Getting fresh air during the day will help both you and your baby sleep better at night, too.

Sweating

During the postpartum period, you may wake up drenched in sweat, but don't worry. This is perfectly normal. It's just another way for your body to get rid of all those extra fluids it has built up during pregnancy.[3] All you can do is adjust your clothing as needed and stay hydrated.

Hair Loss

You may notice you're losing more hair than usual, whether it's while you're brushing or washing your hair. The good news is you're not going to be bald. During pregnancy, your body's hormones have coordinated hair growth. Normally, hairs fall out at different times, but when you're pregnant, they do this in sync. After giving birth, it's time for your hair to fall out. This too shall pass.

Incontinence and/or Constipation

Some women may experience incontinence postpartum. The muscles controlling the flow of urine take quite a beating when you give birth to a baby. However, women who smoke, are obese, give birth to large babies, or had an assisted vaginal delivery (particularly forceps) are more likely to have problems with incontinence. To help with incontinence, you can do regular Kegel exercises.[4] But if it doesn't get better in time, see a doctor.

After giving birth, some women experience constipation. As mentioned earlier, the first bowel movement represents a dreaded, major milestone. Drink plenty of water and stay away from foods, which can constipate you (dairy has that effect), while eating lots of fiber and healthy fats at the same time (fresh fruits are a great idea). Eventually, you'll pass stools and wonder what the big deal was.

Hemorrhoids

Hemorrhoids are something you may still deal with for a while. These like to show up during the last trimester of pregnancy, but they can hang around for a few weeks after giving birth. If you had hemorrhoids during pregnancy, giving birth may have aggravated them, because a lot of pressure was put on your anus during the pushing stage. But since you're already eating plenty of healthy foods and drinking water, those hemorrhoids should go away on their own, given some extra time. In the meantime, warm baths can relieve the pain.

Feeling Blue

Many new mothers experience the baby blues within a few days of giving birth. Lots of things can cause this to happen: changes to your body, fluctuating hormones, trying to adjust to life with a new baby, and more. Sometimes new mothers can feel sad, because they were disappointed with their birth experience, for example, having to have a C-section.

Women can also get depressed because of all the changes they didn't expect. Your body will look nothing like it did before your pregnancy. Besides the new belly fat, you may have horrible stretch marks and leaky breasts and possibly a torn vagina. Some of these things may never go away (stretch marks only fade), but somehow, we learn to adjust. Most of these changes are temporary, and we need to make ourselves aware of that. Other reasons women can become depressed include all the overwhelming responsibilities which come with having a newborn. Especially a first-time mother will feel inadequate, at least some of the time.

To help you get over the baby blues, take naps during the day. I know it's difficult, but you just need to ignore the mess in your house as much as you can. It will still be there for you later. It's time to accept help. Not only does your partner need to learn how to load the dishwasher, but the next time your mother offers to come and help you, let her be useful. She can do laundry, clean the bathroom, or even watch the baby while you take a nap for an hour or two. You may take care of it all by yourself, but your life will be so much easier if you let other people help you.

Don't plan on having time to yourself for the first few months of your baby's life. Don't expect to spring-clean your house or accomplish any other major projects, either. Otherwise, you'll be disappointed when you can't ever seem to get around to doing them. It's perfectly normal to do nothing but take care of your new baby. That's the most important thing you can and should be doing right now. Everything else is secondary.

Unfulfilled expectations may contribute to the baby blues. You daydreamed about life with a baby, but you never imagined having a baby who won't stop crying, no matter what you do. You didn't foresee leaky diapers or the baby vomiting all over you and your bed. These things are part of life with a new baby, more often than we like them to be. But you just need to focus on the good times and enjoy them. Your baby will grow up quickly and make this stage seem like a blur.

Usually, the baby blues come and go on their own. But if you constantly feel down, and the feeling doesn't lessen or go away within two or three weeks of giving birth, please **seek professional help**. Some women experience severe postpartum depression and need medication to get better. And while postpartum depression is less common for homebirthers[5], nobody is exempt. It's okay to have postpartum depression, and it's definitely okay to seek help. **If you ever feel the desire to harm yourself or your baby, you need to get help immediately.**

Life with a Newborn

A new mother is easily swayed by the sheer amount of advice she receives. Unfortunately, a new mother is more likely to listen to expert opinions than her own intuition, because she doesn't yet realize she's the expert on her own baby. **Nobody else knows your baby better than you.** Your baby looks to you to take care of him, and you'll find the strength and ability to do so, because that's what moms do.

Having a baby and raising her is a wonderful journey you're about to embark upon. Pregnancy and childbirth are monumental events, but they pale compared to the many years you'll spend taking care of and worrying about your children. For a smooth start to life with your newborn baby, I've listed a few of the most important topics to help you through the first few days and weeks of your baby's life.

Why Not to Circumcise

Even women who want to have a natural childbirth may still choose to circumcise their baby boy. I know mothers who were against circumcision, but in the end, they allowed their partners to decide. Apparently, it was not worth the battle to them. Even partners who normally want to hear all the pros and cons for an issue can be set on circumcision, especially if they were circumcised themselves.

I hope you make this decision together with your partner. Just because he has a penis doesn't mean he alone knows what's best for your baby boy. But whenever you bring up the subject of circumcision, you need to realize this is a delicate topic. If your partner was circumcised, he may feel inadequate or incomplete. Therefore, you may not want to mention the words 'genital mutilation' in a discussion with him.

I think you have to fight for your baby's right to keep his body the way he was born. It's his by right. Just know, you often only need one parent's consent for the procedure. Therefore, make sure your partner agrees with you.

Circumcising a baby is wrong for several reasons. It's ethically wrong to cut off a part of his penis for no reason at all. The foreskin fulfills several important functions. If it wasn't needed, then boys would be born without it. If your son wanted to be circumcised, he could decide to do it later in life. But it's unfair to make an irreversible decision like this for him when he is too young to make his opinion known. And your baby would tell you no, if he could, because circumcision:

- Is painful
- Is unnecessary
- Reduces sexual pleasure for both the man and the woman
- Can cause complications (1 in 500) and even death (1 in 500,000)

If you want to learn more about circumcision, I recommend you read "The Case Against Circumcision" by Paul M. Fleiss, M.D., which was published in 1997 in the Mothering Journal. You can find the article in full online: http://www.mothersagainstcirc.org/fleiss.html.

189

Originally, circumcision was performed to prevent masturbation. Its obvious use was to diminish sexual pleasure, and it was done to punish boys for masturbating. During the cold war era, private-sector hospitals institutionalized routine circumcision, because it was profitable. In the 1970s, several lawsuits forced hospitals to get the parents' consent for the procedure. This caused the medical profession to invent medical reasons for circumcising boy babies.

Contrary to popular belief, **circumcision is neither healthy nor hygienic**. One of the many functions of the foreskin is to protect. When the foreskin is removed, the body parts which were internal become external. Even after the wound heals, the head of the penis is exposed to urine, feces, and other chemicals, where an uncircumcised penis would have been protected.

The foreskin protects the penis similar to how your eyelids protect your eyes. Females have a foreskin, too. It's called the clitoral hood, and it covers the clitoris. There are some cultures who still mutilate this part as well, either to reduce sexual pleasure or to improve its appearance. In the United States, this has been done in the past. Fortunately, it has since been recognized as an abusive procedure. Hopefully, it's only a matter of a short time until circumcision of boys is discontinued for the same reasons.

When you circumcise your child, you not only expose him to harm, but you also severely diminish his future sex life. Intercourse is more pleasurable for both men and women when the foreskin stays intact. The foreskin is much more sensitive to temperature and texture changes. It's as sensitive as your fingertips or your lips. Once it's removed, millions of nerve endings are gone with it.

There isn't a single medical organization that endorses circumcision. Unfortunately, it's more than an unnecessary procedure, because it's harmful. It can even interfere with your ability to bond with your baby. The pain experienced during circumcision can cause the baby's withdrawal into prolonged un-restful non-REM sleep. In some cases, it can lead to a hemorrhage of the infant or even death.

From an ethical standpoint, you're violating a patient's right by making this decision for your baby. Do you remember reading about informed consent? Your baby is not old enough to make a decision like this, and you're doing it for him. This is okay and necessary during an illness or medical emergency, but circumcision falls under neither one of those categories. It also violates The Hippocratic Oath every doctor has to take: First, do no harm. Babies are helpless and need our protection. They don't need us to hand them over to get cut.

Fortunately, caring for your uncircumcised son is easy. Bathing your son in plain water is the only thing you need to do. Otherwise, his penis is best left alone. The foreskin itself is not retractable until the time is right, and this will not be for several years after your son is out of diapers. And by then, he should be the only one to decide who touches his foreskin.

Breastfeeding

Your baby won't need any other nourishment than what your body is already prepared to feed her. Breastmilk has all the nutrients your baby needs, and it even changes as your baby grows. Your breastmilk doesn't even stay the same during one feeding. The hind milk (what your baby receives at the end of a feeding) is believed to be much fattier to fill your baby's tummy.

To promote breastfeeding from the start, take advantage of the first hour of your baby's life. You can still breastfeed if your baby doesn't get to nurse right away, but the odds are much better if she latches on within the first hour of being born. The key thing you need to pay attention to is your baby's position during nursing: your baby's chest, belly, and knees should touch your abdomen. Your baby needs to face the nipple, and her ear, shoulder, and hip should form a straight line.

Initially, it will seem like you don't really have much milk to give, but your baby is receiving a lot of nutrition from colostrum. Colostrum is the milk your breasts have been producing during your pregnancy. If you've experienced leakage before birth, it was likely colostrum.

After a day or two of colostrum feedings, your milk will come in. It may happen overnight, and then you wake up soaked in the morning. If this is your first baby, your breasts may produce a lot of milk, making it kind of painful. Full breasts can feel rock-solid.

Many people recommend pumping to relieve the pressure and pain, but this can set up a vicious cycle of overproduction. Anytime your baby nurses, your body is told to produce more breastmilk, and pumping sends the same signal. After a few days, your body will regulate itself and produce milk in smaller amounts. But if you pump, your body will ramp up its milk production, thinking demand is up, when in fact the opposite is true.

An icepack on your breasts can help with painful swelling. And even though you're no longer pregnant, you probably still won't get to sleep on your stomach if your breasts are full and aching.

Your baby should empty one breast at each feeding before you offer the second one. You can usually feel a noticeable difference. And yes, this might make your breasts kind of lopsided for a while, but no one will notice. You want your baby to empty one breast to get the rich hind milk. At the next feeding, have your baby nurse on the other side first. Once your baby gets bigger and your breasts adjust their milk volume, she will probably nurse on both sides during each feeding. You still have to switch the beginning sides for each feeding to keep your milk supply fairly even in both breasts.

There are a few ways to accomplish this if you have a hard time remembering which side is next: You can use a bracelet and switch the hand that is wearing it after each nursing session. You could use a paperclip in your bra or whatever other ingenious idea you can come up with. You may develop a favorite nursing side, but don't let it deter you from switching sides at every feeding. Of course, you can make an exception to this rule at night. There's no reason to wake up and switch sides if you and your baby are comfortably co-sleeping and nursing all night long.

While you're breastfeeding, there are still a few things you shouldn't eat, because everything will affect your baby. Caffeine is still a no-no, as are alcoholic beverages. There may even be some foods your baby shows an unfavorable reaction to. For example, you may notice that she is gassy or has a bad diaper rash. Try to eliminate certain foods from your diet to see if it helps. Babies are usually fine with you eating spicy foods if they were used to them in the uterus, but sometimes babies show a reaction to dairy in the mother's diet. Other times, they may not tolerate certain fruits or vegetables. You'll just have to experiment with what you eat and find out what works best for the two of you.

There's no need to start your baby on solid foods until he's at least six months old. You can wait a lot longer if you want. My boys didn't show any interest in food until they were almost a year old. Babies thrive on breastmilk alone. Even on warm days, they don't need water. Actually, giving water to a newborn baby can be dangerous. But if it's hot, then you need to nurse often enough for them to stay hydrated.

As mentioned before, a tongue tie or lip tie can seriously impede breastfeeding. If your baby doesn't suckle well or long enough, he may not be capable of nursing properly because of a tie. Tongue ties can vary in severity and aren't always obvious. Here's a list of signs your baby may have a tongue tie:

- Poor latch
- Painful nursing sessions
- Constant hunger
- Frustration with nursing

- Reflux or spitting up
- Milk leaking out of baby's mouth
- Clicking or smacking noises
- Poor weight gain

For any problems with breastfeeding (whether related to a tongue tie or not), it's a good idea to reach out to a lactation consultant. If you suspect a tongue tie, check the specialist's credentials, as many doctors simply aren't trained to diagnose or treat them.

Diapering

After the first few days when the meconium disappears, your baby's stools will have a light brown, mustard color. Breastfed babies are rarely ever constipated, and it can be normal for them not to have a bowel movement every day. As long as your baby is eating and peeing regularly and not straining without results, she's probably just fine. In fact, some breastfed babies can go for as long as two weeks without a bowel movement.

When selecting which type of diapers to use, you may feel overwhelmed. If you decide on disposable diapers, it may be worth getting a membership at Costco or Sam's Club or purchase store-brand diapers at your local grocery store. Expect to use a lot of diapers. Try out different kinds to see which ones you like best, because some diapers fit better than others.

If you're interested in using cloth diapers, you'll probably still need to do some research beforehand. First, there are pre-fold cloth diapers, which is what our parent's generation was using. The pre-fold cloth diaper looks like a rectangle. When you use it, you have to fold it specially to fit the baby, and then it needs to get secured with pins. Nowadays, instead of pins, you can buy snappy devices aptly called cloth diaper fasteners. These fasteners work by grasping onto the fabric. By the way, folding the pre-fold diapers is easy once you've done it a couple of times. For extra protection, you can use plastic pants which just get pulled over the cloth diaper. This will keep your baby's clothes dry.

If you plan on using elimination communication, you won't need a lot of diapers at all. You can get a few pre-fold cloth diapers to prevent misses, but you probably won't need the plastic pants, unless you're out and about and cannot pay attention to your baby's signals.

Instead of pre-fold cloth diapers, you can also purchase all-in-one cloth diapers. They are much more expensive than the pre-fold kind, but they look a lot like a disposable diaper. They're already the right shape, and they use snaps or Velcro to tighten. Snaps are used to adjust sizing. These diapers have a waterproof layer on the outside, and they use cloth inserts on the inside to absorb the moisture. You can use pre-fold diapers as inserts for some all-in-one diapers.

While all-in-one cloth diapers present quite an upfront investment, you'll save a lot of money down the road compared to disposable diapers. Cloth diapers are better for the environment, and they're nicer to your baby's bottom, too. If you don't like the price tag of new cloth diapers, consider buying used ones. Since they usually last through several babies, buying used cloth diapers is a valid option.

Newborns aren't anywhere near as squirmy as older babies. Therefore, this is a perfect time to practice diapering if you have little or no experience with it. Older babies often resent being laid down to get diapered, especially once they become mobile. But by then, you'll be a pro.

When you diaper your baby, lay her on a waterproof surface. This way, you'll protect your carpet, your bed, and your furniture from accidents. For a boy, lay a diaper over him since his pee can be harder to contain. And obviously, don't leave your baby unattended on a changing table, because you don't want him to roll off.

As you're cleaning your baby, always wipe front to back, especially for little girls. And even boys need to be wiped after they pee,

195

because they sit in the wet diaper for at least a few minutes until you can change them.

For wipes, you have the option of disposable or cloth. Disposable wipes use a lot of chemicals (even the hypoallergenic ones), and it may be nicer to your baby's bottom to use cloth if you can. This means more laundry for you, but greater savings in the long run. It's easier to put both diapers and wipes in the laundry together than to put them in separate bins. If you're using disposable diapers, you can use wet paper towels instead of chemical wipes. Just add water and start wiping.

Finally, you need to decide what you want to do about diaper rashes. While you can buy a variety of diaper rash crèmes at the store, they may not be what you want. Personally, I have found coconut oil to be very effective. But it's not a good idea to use crèmes and lotions with several unpronounceable ingredients on your baby's skin, because your baby's skin is extremely absorbent. For diaper rashes, letting your baby be butt-naked a few times throughout the day may accomplish more than any diaper rash crème could.

Bathing

Babies don't need baths every day. In fact, you should hold off on bathing your baby. Your baby is born with a protective cover on his skin, and you don't want to wash this off too soon. You can spot clean where he's poopy or bloody after birth, but there's no need to put the baby in the tub. It's safest to wait until the umbilical cord falls off. Until then, you can give your baby a sponge bath.

When you're ready to give your baby his first bath, be careful to support his head. Initially, it's nice to have someone available to help, because wet babies are really slippery. And this way, you can take some pictures. Your newborn baby may not like baths in the beginning. But when your baby gets older, he'll probably love playing in the water.

When you clean your baby, get into all the creases around his neck, under his arms, and behind his ears. Don't forget to pay attention to the genitals. A sponge bath may actually result in a cleaner baby, because it's difficult to hold a newborn baby in the tub while trying to clean him at the same time. After the bath, wrap him up in a towel to keep him warm. And pay special attention to his head since this is where all the heat escapes. You can put a hat on him until he's warmed up.

Umbilical Care

You don't need to use alcohol to clean the umbilical stump. A clean, wet washcloth will do it, and once the stump falls off partially, you can get underneath it with a Q-Tip[6]. Keep the umbilical area dry and clean at all times, until the stump falls off, which usually happens after a week or two.

The umbilical stump rarely bothers babies at all, and you can still dress and diaper her. Just fold the diaper to fit it under the cord stump. This way, her navel doesn't get soiled. You can even buy disposable newborn diapers with a cutout for the umbilical cord.

When the umbilical cord falls off, you may see a bit of bleeding, or you may find dried blood around the belly button. Small amounts of blood can be normal, but if it doesn't stop bleeding after you put pressure on it, then you need to take your baby to a doctor as soon as possible.

How to Get a Birth Certificate

One of the many challenges of giving birth unassisted is getting a birth certificate for your baby. While you're technically not required to get a birth certificate, things are going to be more difficult without one. A birth certificate is usually necessary to get a Social Security number, a driver's license, a passport, and a marriage license. The longer you wait, the more difficult it may be to prove the birth of your child to the authorities that issue birth certificates.

From personal experience, I can say getting a birth certificate isn't always easy. But how difficult it really is depends on the state you live in, the clerk you're dealing with, and what kind of (medical) records you have. Each state has its own process, and therefore I can't tell you exactly what you need to do. However, there are a few things you can do to make things easier for yourself.

1. Get an official pregnancy test done before you give birth and keep a record of it. You can have this done at your general practitioner.
2. Research the laws for your state.
3. Reach out to online communities for advice from other moms in your state.
4. Consider taking your baby to a doctor for an exam to establish a medical record. This doesn't need to happen right after birth—you can wait a few days.
5. Find someone other than your partner who will attest to having knowledge of your pregnancy and birth.

I've given birth unassisted in Utah and in Texas. Both states required proof of pregnancy and proof the infant was born alive and born on the date stated. Additionally, I had to provide proof of residency, because the baby was born at home.

While it's easy to make a copy of your utility bill, it's not as easy to get proof of your pregnancy if you choose to do your own prenatal care (or choose not to have any prenatal care at all). Fortunately, you can get a pregnancy test done at a doctor's office without agreeing to additional treatment. The doctor I chose was just a general practitioner, so there was never a question of seeking prenatal care with her.

While laws can change, it's not likely for the rules on reporting non-institutional births to change often. You can ask other women who've given birth unassisted in your state for advice (as of this writing, I recommend searching unassisted childbirth groups on

Facebook). When you're researching how to get a birth certificate, remember **you have to be the one to report the birth**. You can't order a copy of the birth certificate until you have reported the birth to the authorities. However, the place where you would normally order the birth certificate is the same place you contact to report a birth. It's usually called Vital Statistics or Vital Records and found in your county clerk's office.

There are two ways to approach this problem when you're talking to the people who take care of the paperwork. You could talk to them before you have the baby, letting them know what you're planning on doing and how you can make this process easier. Alternatively, you can come in after the fact and hope you can find the documents they require.

Some women choose to hire a midwife and just call her after the fact. Others even go to the hospital within hours of giving birth unassisted, just to not have to worry about the official paperwork. How you want to handle it is totally up to you. However, if you bring a newborn baby to the hospital, you might find doctors and nurses are just itching to administer various newborn procedures you'd rather skip.

Fortunately, you don't have to revise your birth plans for the birth certificate. You have the right to receive one for your baby, even if it takes a while. I highly recommend getting a pregnancy test done at a doctor's office—even if you don't have insurance, it shouldn't cost much and might save you a lot of trouble later. Then I'd suggest calling the local county clerk's office within a few days of the baby's birth to get the ball rolling. If you can give birth unassisted, you can get a birth certificate for your baby.

---

[1] Mayo Foundation for Education and Research (2014). "Postpartum care: What to expect after a vaginal delivery." Retrieved from

http://www.mayoclinic.org/healthy-living/labor-and-delivery/in-depth/postpartum-care/art-20047233?pg=1.

[2] Spiliopoulos, Michail, MD (2013). "Normal and Abnormal Puerperium." Retrieved from http://emedicine.medscape.com/article/260187-overview.

[3] BabyCenter Medical Advisory Board (2014). "Postpartum sweating." Retrieved from http://www.babycenter.com/0_postpartum-sweating_11720.bc.

[4] BabyCenter Medical Advisory Board (2013). "Postpartum urinary incontinence." Retrieved from http://www.babycenter.com/0_postpartum-urinary-incontinence_1152241.bc?page=1.

[5] Bland (2009) Missouri Western State University. "The Effect of Birth Experience on Postpartum Depression". Retrieved from http://clearinghouse.missouriwestern.edu/manuscripts/59.php.

[6] American Pregnancy Association (2011). "Umbilical Cord Care." Retrieved from http://americanpregnancy.org/firstyearoflife/umbilicalcord.htm.

Chapter 6

Father's Guide

Quick List

<u>Labor:</u> Encourage frequent bathroom breaks. Offer drinks often. When mother has an urge to move her bowels, birth is imminent.

<u>Birth:</u> Encourage good positioning of the mother (upright, standing, on all fours). Encourage her to push when she feels the need.

<u>Bag of Water:</u> Labor will probably begin within 48 hours after the bag of waters breaks. If the mother is already in labor, then the breaking of the water can signal the start of baby's birth, or it can happen during birth.

<u>Cord:</u> Leave the umbilical cord alone. Do not pull on it. Wait to cut the cord until it has completely stopped pulsating.

<u>During Birth:</u> Never pull on the baby, whichever position he is in. If the baby's shoulders are stuck (very rare), try to help by turning the baby. Wait for at least two contractions after the head is born to assist. In most cases, the problem resolves itself.

<u>Hand First:</u> This is fine if the hand is near or on top of the head. It can prolong labor and childbirth, but a natural birth is certainly possible. Encourage good positioning and encourage the mother to keep up her strength. If you see no head with the hand, the woman needs to go to the hospital to have a C-section. Giving birth vaginally in this position is impossible.

Cord First: If the cord falls out before the baby is born, and the mother has the urge to push, encourage her to bear down hard to give birth to her baby quickly. Otherwise, get mother in knee-chest position to take the pressure off the cord and get her to the hospital as quickly as possible. Wrap the cord loosely in a warm, wet towel.

Butt or Legs first: Help the mother to her hands and knees or to standing and guard her from falling. **Don't touch the baby.**

Baby not breathing: If the baby is grey or blue and limp, wipe baby's face and then start artificial respiration.

Shock: Woman is pale, sweaty, weak, breathing hard, and thirsty. Keep her cool, on her back, and with her feet up. Give her water with one teaspoon of salt to a quart to drink. Get her to the hospital quickly after a hemorrhage.

Excessive Bleeding: Encourage placenta to be born by massaging the uterus. If excessive bleeding is accompanied by a woman in shock, get her to the hospital quickly.

How to Recognize the Signs of Labor

While there are quite a few early warning signs, it can take some time for the mother or her birth attendant to realize she's in labor. Labor can be accompanied by one or more of the following signs:

- Contractions
- Back pain
- Bloody show
- Diarrhea
- Water breaking

The pregnant woman may experience contractions prior to labor. She may have back pain and diarrhea a few days or weeks before actual labor begins. It's also possible for her water to break several hours or even days before she goes into labor.

Most of the time, a pregnant woman cannot mistake recurring contractions for too long. With true labor, contractions become more regular and intense. Some women don't experience any pain during contractions at all. However, they'll still notice the increasing intensity.

Even though most women don't go into labor until they're anywhere from 37 to 42 weeks along, it's possible for a pregnant woman to go into labor earlier. If the woman is having twins, labor can start significantly sooner. Of course, the earlier babies are born, the more likely it is they'll need medical attention.

For the attendant, it's important to observe the laboring woman closely to gauge how labor is progressing. Her behavior can clue you in. If the woman is having a hard time tolerating the pain, she may be close to giving birth.

As the birth attendant, your role is to encourage the woman to stay calm and keep breathing. Women are meant to give birth, and even though it can be painful, she can handle it. When it becomes seemingly unbearable, it's likely she's almost ready to give birth. Reassure her she's doing great and that every contraction gets her closer to see her baby.

What Supplies to Get Ready

Unless you were already planning a homebirth, you may not have any proper supplies on hand. However, that's not a big problem. If you have access to a few clean towels and a knife or scissors, you're in great shape.

If possible, warm up a few towels in the dryer. These will be necessary to keep the baby warm once he's born. The mother may need a sheet or a blanket to stay warm afterwards, too.

If you can find something to protect the flooring, this will make your life easier afterwards. Otherwise, bloodstains clean up really well using only cold water.

While the woman is in labor, sterilize a pair of scissors or a knife by boiling them in water for a few minutes. You'll use it to cut the umbilical cord later. By the way, cutting the cord doesn't need to happen on a time schedule. The longer you wait with cutting the cord, the better.

Finally, if you're with a laboring woman outside or in a vehicle, you won't have any supplies handy. Instead of a towel, find an extra blanket or item of clothing. If all else fails, use your T-shirt to wrap the baby in. In addition, keep the baby close to the mother after birth to help him regulate his body temperature.

If the baby is born on the go (for example, on the way to the hospital), you can wait until you get to your destination to cut the cord. However, take all necessary steps to ensure baby and mother are comfortable and warm.

How to Assist during Labor

A laboring woman needs little physical assistance. Her body will give birth, regardless of your involvement. If you're dealing with a first-time mother, you may need to offer extra reassurance in the form of soothing encouragement.

Pay attention to the laboring woman. If she asks you to leave her alone, honor her wish, but remain nearby to assist her when necessary.

Your primary job is to ensure the laboring woman is drinking and urinating regularly by periodically offering her water to drink. During the early stages of labor, she may even be hungry.

Encourage the laboring woman to empty her bladder regularly, at least once every hour. A full bladder can impede labor. Emptying the bladder also has the physical side effect of relaxing the muscles relevant during childbirth. However, during the end of the first stage of labor, it may be very uncomfortable for the woman to sit on the toilet during a contraction.

What Happens Next?

You may have little or no experience with the process of childbirth. Therefore, it makes sense to get an overview of the three stages of labor.

First Stage of Labor

The first stage of labor takes the longest of all three stages. That's why it's divided into its own three phases: early labor, active labor, and transition. During the first stage of labor, the contractions help dilate the cervix to 10 cm, at which point the baby will be born.

As a non-medical birth attendant, you won't be checking the woman's dilation. Therefore, you may not notice when she moves from early to active labor or from active labor to transition. Fortunately, this isn't a problem.

During early labor, the laboring woman can still talk, walk around, and pursue an activity with little difficulty. If labor starts at night, it makes sense to get as much rest as possible. Even if sleep is out of the question, the laboring woman shouldn't start doing laundry or cleaning the house.

If labor starts during the daytime, encourage the laboring woman to do whatever she feels like doing. For example, she can read a book, go for a walk, or play a card game. During early labor, contractions are usually far apart and not very painful.

You can time the contractions to assess how things are progressing. However, the demeanor of the laboring woman will change as she enters active labor, and this serves as a better indicator of progress than the clock.

During active labor, contractions will increase in intensity and frequency. The laboring woman concentrates more on breathing through the contractions. Encourage her to breathe calmly. If you notice hyperventilating, breathe deeply with her. You must remain calm even if she isn't.

During transition, the laboring woman may be in a lot of pain. Fortunately, transition doesn't last as long as early or active labor. If the laboring woman feels like giving up or crying, it's your job as the birth attendant to reassure her. Keep offering her water throughout her entire labor. You can also provide her with conversation if she so desires.

Some women prefer to be alone, but others may like the distraction company provides. Pay attention to what she wants. And if she's short with you, don't take it personally.

Second Stage of Labor

During the second stage of labor, the baby is born. The birth of a baby rarely takes long, especially compared to the first stage of labor.

At the end of transition, the laboring woman will most likely experience an incredible urge to push. She might actually mistake it for the need to move her bowels.

Without a medical attendant present, always leave the mother in charge. Encourage her to get in a position conducive to pushing, for example, standing, squatting, or on her hands and knees. The laboring woman should not lie on her back to give birth. Not only does the woman have to work against gravity, but her pelvis cannot open as much as in a different position. Most women will naturally gravitate towards a suitable position, but they may also move around and switch positions.

If the woman has the urge to push, she may do so, but only when she feels the need. It may take several pushes for the baby to be born. If the woman has had a baby before, the pushing stage probably won't last long.

Most babies are born head first. It's possible for the baby to be born butt first. In rare cases, you may see feet or hands first. The woman should labor in a position that allows gravity to help. For a breech birth, it's extremely important for the woman to be standing, squatting, or on all fours.

If the baby is born breech, never attempt to pull on the baby. Instead, help the woman to a squatting or standing position. The head won't be stuck for long, and the next contraction or two should get the baby out.

Once the baby is born, you can place the baby in his mother's arms and cover both with a warm towel or blanket. If possible, write down what time the baby was born. But first, make sure baby and mother are alert and well.

Third Stage of Labor

During the third stage of labor, the placenta is born. This is neither painful nor difficult for the laboring woman. Once her baby is born, pain is a thing of the past. While there may be bleeding, it should be light. Keep a close eye on the mother. If she experiences light-headedness or dizziness, it may be a sign of too much blood loss.

While the placenta should be born in one piece, there's no rush for this to happen. Never pull on the umbilical cord.

If it has been more than an hour, and you're getting worried about the placenta, there are a few things to try. Sometimes, the placenta is just resting in the vagina. It will come out easily as soon as the woman switches positions. The mother should nurse her baby.

Breastfeeding releases oxytocin, which encourages contractions and can help the placenta along.

If all else fails, press down on the woman's uterus to encourage it to shrink. It should be right around her belly button. This will be painful to her. Therefore, don't do this unless it's necessary.

Cheat Sheets

How to Assist during Labor

1. Remind the laboring woman to go to the bathroom at least once every hour.
2. Offer the laboring woman water to drink. Since she'll probably just take a sip at a time, keep offering it to her every 10 minutes. It helps if the cup has a straw so you can hold it for her.
3. If the woman wants to give up, offer her gentle encouragement.
4. If she has a really hard time, offer to help her into the tub or the shower. Make sure the tub is not slippery and help her sit down.
5. You can talk to the laboring woman, but if she asks you to be quiet, abide by her wishes.
6. If you're comfortable with it, offer a massage or other physical contact. Some women really crave touch, while others prefer to be left alone.

How to Assist during the Birth

1. Encourage the woman to be in a favorable position. Don't let her lie on her back.
2. Let her scream if she feels like it (some women are screamers, some aren't). Don't worry about the neighbors.
3. Have warm towels ready if she's actively pushing.
4. Make sure the baby is caught or lands safely.
5. Don't pull on the umbilical cord.

6. Help her hold her baby to keep mother and baby warm.

How to Evaluate the Baby

1. The baby needs to breathe within the first minute of being born. Encourage this by gently wiping mucus off the baby's face and rubbing his back. Suctioning nose and mouth isn't usually necessary.
2. Slightly elevating the baby's body and rubbing the baby's back and flicking his feet may help him breathe on his own. If not, place the infant on his tummy with his head to the side to allow the mucus to drain. As a last resort, mouth-to-mouth resuscitation should be tried.
3. The baby's color should perk up within a few minutes.
4. The baby needs nothing except to be held and loved, at least for the first little while.

How to Evaluate the Mother

1. Monitor the mother after the birth. If she shows signs of dizziness, shock, extreme blood loss or any other problems, you'll need to call for help.
2. After the baby is born, the mother won't feel any pain at all. She will most likely feel relieved, elated, and emotional. Let her hold her baby. She needs it as much as the baby does.

The Cord and the Placenta

1. There's no rush the cut the cord. Don't cut it until it stops pulsating.
2. There's no immediate rush to birth the placenta. Allow mother and baby to bond and nurse, and it will happen.
3. If the placenta hasn't been born after an hour or more, encourage the woman to switch positions. She can try to push it out, but you should never tug on the cord. Breastfeeding her new baby will release oxytocin and make the uterus contract. This can speed up the delivery of the placenta. You can also try massaging or pressing down on the

uterus through the belly if needed—this is a last resort option.

4. Don't place the placenta into the regular trash, because it might invite unnecessary attention. If you don't want to encapsulate it, bury it outside.

5. Tie off the cord with shoestring within six inches away from your baby's belly. Tie it off again another inch or two from there and then use scissors to cut in the middle. Later, after the baby has nursed, when you're ready to weigh him, use a clamp to shorten the umbilical cord attached to his belly.

6. The placenta should be in one piece with no torn parts. You should be able to locate three twists in the placenta (three arteries and one vein).

The First Few Days after Birth

1. The new baby should nurse frequently. Even before the milk comes in, the baby will get plenty of nutrients from the mother's colostrum. What goes in must come out. If you're changing diapers a lot, you probably have nothing to worry about.

2. The mother may experience severe cramping after birth. This is completely normal. The uterus is shrinking, and this can be painful, especially after second and subsequent births. The mother can try a hot pillow, massage, switching positions, and over-the-counter Ibuprofen. The afterpains may be worse during nursing sessions.

3. If you haven't done the research already, figure out how to get a birth certificate for your baby.

Dealing with Complications

When to Seek Medical Attention

- Sharp pains that are not labor contractions
- Excessive blood loss of the mother

- Cord prolapse (the umbilical cord comes out first with no baby in sight)
- Fever
- Postpartum hemorrhage
- Retained placenta
- Newborn who can't maintain temperature
- Newborn anomalies

When in Doubt, Do Nothing

The most important advice anyone can give a birth attendant is to do nothing at all. Most likely, the birth will proceed on its own with no intervention on your part. In fact, you can cause more harm if you interfere unnecessarily. That being said, there are a few cases in which the birth attendant can make a positive difference for the outcome of the birth.

Breech Baby

If you suspect a breech baby, don't panic. It's highly likely nothing will go wrong. Ensure the woman is laboring in a suitable position: standing or on all fours. This will help her birth the baby safely. With a breech baby, the head will be born last. Whatever you do, do not pull on or touch the baby! Otherwise, you'll hurt him, and you might even cause his death.

After the baby's body is out, you may feel eager for the head to be born. If the head is not born within two more contractions, you can use your fingers to create an opening for the baby to breathe. Don't pull on the head and don't try to get him out. Instead, make sure the baby can receive oxygen. If the baby is stuck, have the laboring woman change positions, if possible. If all else fails, call for help.

Baby Stuck during Birth

Most babies are born head first. But if the baby's head is out and the next two contractions do not deliver the rest of the baby, the baby's shoulders may be stuck. Encourage the mother to change positions. This alone may be enough to get the baby "unstuck".

If all else fails, you can rotate the baby by hooking a finger under the arm of the baby and gently pulling it towards the baby's face. The shoulder may just be stuck behind the mother's pubic bone. You need to be careful when you do this as to not hurt the baby or the mother.

Cord around the Baby's Neck

It happens often that the umbilical cord is wrapped around the baby's head, sometimes more than once and often rather tightly. This is not necessarily a cause for concern. Once the baby is born, it's easy to unwind the cord without causing any trouble.

When the Hand Comes First

While it's not common, it's absolutely possible for the baby to have her hands on or near her head. There's no reason to panic. While some midwives might feel the hand near the baby's head through the mother's abdomen, this is not something they usually look for. In an ultrasound, this would be easily apparent.

If the baby's hand is near or on his head, labor and birth will probably take longer than normal. Therefore, keep the laboring mother motivated, hydrated, and fed throughout the entire process.

If you notice the baby's hand at the vaginal opening with no sign of his head, then that's a sign the baby is in an impossible position. The chances of a baby lying sideways (transverse) like this are really slim. It's more likely to happen when there are multiple babies, a low-lying placenta, or other issues with the uterus or the baby.

If the baby is in such a position, get the woman to the hospital. The only way for the baby to be born is via C-section. If the position of the baby is known before labor, there's a chance an experienced physician or midwife can turn him.

When the Cord Comes First

If the umbilical cord falls out of the vagina alone, wrap it up loosely in a warm, moist towel. This condition is rare but serious. It's called umbilical cord prolapse. If the woman has the urge to push, she should bear down as hard and quickly as possible. If the woman doesn't have the urge to push, take her to the hospital immediately.

The umbilical cord is the only source of oxygen for the baby. The cord must never be pulled on, and it can't be compressed. To protect the baby, ask the woman to get on her knees with her chest on the floor to relieve the pressure on the cord. In this position, she needs to be taken to the hospital as soon as possible.

Face First

Most head presentations don't pose additional difficulties during labor. For example, a baby may be born face first. If the baby is in this position, the mother may experience strong back labor. But until the baby is born, you won't know for sure which way the head is facing. After such a birth, the baby's face may be swollen, but this should improve within a few hours after birth.

Helping Baby Breathe

Sometimes, babies need a little help breathing at birth. While most babies will breathe and cry on their own shortly after being born, some don't. You can wipe the baby's face with a clean cloth to start with.

If wiping the baby's face doesn't show satisfactory results, put the baby on his tummy with his head facing to the side. This will allow the mucus to drain. His feet should be slightly elevated above his head. In this position, you can stroke the baby's back and flick his feet to encourage him to start breathing.

You must handle a newborn baby gently. You can perform mouth-to-mouth artificial respiration until the baby can breathe without assistance. Use small puffs of air in one-second intervals. As a last resort, you can try CPR. For this, the infant needs to lie on his back on a flat, firm surface. Use two or three fingers to compress the chest (30 compressions) and then give two rescue breaths with your mouth by covering the baby's mouth and nose. You need to repeat this until the baby breathes on his own or until emergency personnel take over. Most likely, you won't have to administer CPR.

Premature Baby

If the baby is born prematurely, the primary concern after proper breathing is the baby's ability to maintain his body temperature. The best way to keep the baby warm and help him regulate his temperature is to keep him skin-to-skin with his mother with a warm towel or blanket over both of them. Depending on how early the baby was born, it's possible for him to have other health problems as well. Observe the newborn baby closely and get him medical attention if necessary.

Twins

Twins are born in the same way as a single baby. It's possible for at least one of them to be born in a breech position. Twins also tend to be born earlier during pregnancy. Therefore, one or both of them might need medical attention if they are very premature.

It's possible for a woman to go into labor without knowing she's having twins. However, she will be much bigger than a mother with only one baby. Twins are full-term at 37 weeks, but mothers of twins often go into labor sooner. When twins are born past 32 to 34 weeks of gestation, they have an excellent chance of survival. However, they may still need oxygen to help them breathe if their lungs aren't fully developed.[1]

Hemorrhage

The mother may hemorrhage before the birth. An early separation of the placenta from the wall of the womb can be the cause. A hemorrhage before birth indicates a need for medical help. The bleeding may be profuse and occur repeatedly. If this is the case, take the mother to the hospital right away for appropriate medical attention.

Hemorrhages after birth are more common than hemorrhages before birth. That being said, a hemorrhage is still not a likely event to happen.

In the event of a hemorrhage after the baby is born, help the placenta along if it hasn't been born already. While it can take some time for the placenta to appear, you can speed it up by massaging the uterus through the abdominal wall. Once the uterus becomes hard, you can use gentle downward pressure to press out the placenta. Keep the pressure within the limits of the woman's comfort.

Dealing with Blood Loss

It's natural for the woman to lose a lot of blood right after giving birth. And while it may seem like a lot of blood at once, the bleeding stops fairly quickly. The amount of blood loss is less than two cups' worth for a natural childbirth. Keep in mind it may look like a lot more if the woman gives birth in the water.

If you're not adept at estimating blood loss, pay attention to the behavior of the mother. If there are any signs of shock (see below), she will need to be treated at the hospital for postpartum hemorrhage.

Treatment of Shock

A woman who has hemorrhaged will have other symptoms besides blood loss. She will be in shock. She will have chilly, sweaty, and/or pale skin, be breathing heavily, or be feeling excessively thirsty and weak. You need to keep the woman lying down, preferably with her feet up. A hemorrhage must be treated as an emergency. Get the woman to the hospital as quickly as possible. Hemorrhages aren't necessarily fatal as long as they're treated promptly.

Miscarriage

A miscarriage happens usually during early pregnancy. There is nothing the attendant can do in this case. The woman will pass blood clots for a while. If the bleeding is excessive, get her to the hospital. But most likely, the miscarriage will take its course without additional help from anyone else.

---

[1] What to Expect (n.d.). "Your Tentative Timetable" Retrieved from http://www.whattoexpect.com/pregnancy/twins-and-multiples/giving-birth/your-tentative-timetable.aspx.

Final Words

Did this book help you prepare for your homebirth?

Please take a moment and **rate or review** *The Unassisted Baby* at the retailer you've purchased it from.

I hope this book has helped resolve some of your concerns about unassisted pregnancy and childbirth. There are other great reads on natural childbirth, some of which you can find in the list of resources following this chapter.

For me, giving birth unassisted was amazing and life-changing. Going through an unassisted pregnancy and birth was even more empowering. I actually enjoyed my second and third unassisted births even more because I had learned to have faith in myself.

I would enjoy hearing from you if you want to share your birth story, your thoughts about planning an unassisted birth, or questions about the book. Please send an email to email@anitaevensen.com.

Finally, come and check out my website for more information on unassisted pregnancy and childbirth as well as printable cheat sheets:

www.TheUnassistedBaby.com

Happy Birthing!

My Pregnancy and Childbirth Experiences

First Pregnancy
(Hospital Birth with an OB/GYN)

My first daughter was born 'conventionally' in a hospital in 2005. During the pregnancy, I received regular prenatal care. The only thing I refused was a flu shot. Otherwise, I pretty much went along with whatever the doctor prescribed.

I gained plenty of weight, but unfortunately, my baby did not gain enough. After various ultrasounds showed the baby wasn't growing as much as she should, the doctor asked me to come into the office twice a week. Each visit included a fetal non-stress test to check on the baby.

The doctor wanted to induce labor by 37 weeks, unless fetal monitoring indicated the need for an even sooner delivery. He said my baby wasn't growing enough and would do better outside the womb. The constant doctor visits during my pregnancy worried me. The only other thing my OB/GYN recommended was for me to drink Boost. While it may have helped me gain more weight, it certainly didn't help my baby.

Another stressful factor during the pregnancy was the fact that my husband wasn't around. He was a submariner in the U.S. Navy. He was out to sea and would have returned in time for my due date, but our baby decided she couldn't wait. He did not get to see her until she was already over a week old, because at 36 weeks and 2 days my water broke.

I didn't know that's what it was. It was just a slow, constant trickle, and in my ignorance, I thought it was urine. Two days later, I had an appointment for the fetal non-stress test again. During an ultrasound, the doctor noticed my amniotic fluid was low. I told him about the urine leaking, but he knew right away it was my water. He promptly sent me to the hospital to be induced. I was in disbelief in the waiting room and throughout the entire labor. Part of me really thought my husband would show up at any moment.

Nobody checked my cervix again, because of the ruptured membranes. They gave me Pitocin, and I eventually received an epidural during transition, only to give birth to my first baby 30 minutes afterwards. I wasn't alone during the birth. One of my friends and my mother-in-law were there to welcome my baby into the world with me, but neither thought getting an epidural was a big deal.

For a first baby, labor went pretty fast. After checking into the hospital without contractions, it only took three or four hours until my daughter was born. My doctor barely had time to put his gloves on to catch my baby. Baby Melanie weighed 4 pounds, which is small, even considering her gestational age. The nurses took her immediately to weigh her while I received stitches for my tears. When I look back at it, I can't believe I tore for a 4-pound baby. But at the time, it didn't even occur to me this wasn't the natural order of things. After my baby was examined, prodded, cleaned up, dressed, and swaddled, they allowed me to hold her.

Even though I didn't know what to do, she had no problems nursing. She even received a pacifier from well-meaning nurses against my wishes. I was told to supplement her feedings with a bottle, because she was so small. In the first few days of her life, my daughter went from bottle to breast without any problems. They diagnosed her with jaundice, and she had to spend some time under the bilirubin lights.

I'm still aching for the kind of birth I didn't have with her. I wish things had been different. Fortunately, we had a wonderful breastfeeding relationship. I nursed her for her entire first year. And even though it took me several weeks to truly bond with her, I love her like every mother loves her child.

I felt disappointed with the birth, because I didn't want to have an epidural. The perineal tear and the stitches never bothered me until much later. Looking back on it, I'm not surprised I tore. I was pushing on my back while I was numb from the epidural. Therefore, I didn't know how much pressure I was putting on my perineum by pushing, since I couldn't feel anything.

Maybe I had to have a birth like this to want something different the next time around.

Second Pregnancy
(Birth Center Birth with a Midwife)

Throughout my second pregnancy, I had four different caregivers. Initially, I saw the same doctor I had with my first, but then we moved. My husband was still in the Navy. His new duty station had a military hospital on base, which I had to go to. The horror stories told by his coworkers and others did little to help the hospital's reputation. And while I had an ultrasound done at the base hospital, I switched providers after only one prenatal appointment.

I went to a civilian doctor upon a friend's recommendation. He immediately classified my pregnancy as high-risk, because I had given birth to a low-weight, pre-term baby before. He ordered excessive ultrasound monitoring from the beginning. I didn't feel comfortable asking him questions, and I also didn't trust him to hold off on interventions. When I thought about his highly medical approach, I started reading up on natural childbirth, because this was something I still really wanted.

At first, my husband was nervous about giving birth anywhere other than at a hospital. However, in time, he came around after I talked to him about the harm of interventions, and how they can hinder the natural process of birth.

I found a birth center with two wonderful midwives. I was impressed by how much time they spent talking to me during appointments. I liked that they gave me the ability to opt out of medical interventions long before my due date, such as the antibiotic eye ointment and the Vitamin K shot.

After I passed my due date, I became anxious. The midwives tried to reassure me and said women rarely go past 42 weeks. However, if I was still pregnant at 42 weeks, I would have to give birth at the hospital.

I really didn't want to go to the hospital. Therefore, I consented to a membrane sweep eight days after my due date. Two days later, I woke up with contractions. I paced the house all morning and eventually gave the midwives a call. One of them agreed to meet me at the birth center to check my progress. My husband drove me there after we dropped off our daughter at the babysitter's house.

Baby Becky was born in the water at the birth center, ten days after her due date. The midwife caught the baby and promptly placed her on my chest. It was a wonderful feeling to hold the baby against my skin. After a little while, I moved from the tub to the bed. In hindsight, I remember my midwife lightly tugged on the umbilical cord to get the placenta out. Now I know she shouldn't have done that, because it could have made the placenta rupture. After the placenta was delivered, she stitched me up. I remember the needle hurt, because it was impossible to numb the area completely.

About two hours after the birth, my husband drove me and our newborn daughter home. I felt much better than after the first birth. The hospital birth had left me feeling weak. I had left in a wheelchair after staying there for five days. That's why I was amazed I could walk and function normally right after giving birth this time. Our baby weighed a healthy 8 pounds and 4 ounces, more than twice the size of my first.

Giving birth in a birth center with the midwife present definitely opened up a new perspective on childbirth for me. I felt I could handle labor, the contractions, and the pain during the pushing phase quite well. I felt euphoric for weeks after giving birth. I felt like I was in charge, although looking back, I can see this wasn't necessarily true. The midwife and a student midwife instructed me when to push, and while they knew I could give birth to this baby without medical interventions, they didn't believe I could give birth on my own. And at the time, I probably wasn't ready for that.

Third Pregnancy (Miscarriage)

My third pregnancy ended in a miscarriage. I had engaged a different midwife (we had moved to a different state) for the pregnancy, but at six weeks, it was too early to check for a heartbeat. I had bled throughout the pregnancy and was worried about it. The midwife told me there was not much to do but wait and see.

At nine weeks, I started having cramps (kind of like a bad period) and passed blood clots all night long. The midwife told me on the phone what I already knew: this baby would not be born. My body had no issues getting rid of the evidence. Cramping and bleeding were my only physical symptoms. I didn't get evaluated by anyone during the miscarriage or afterwards. I felt there wasn't really any need for it, and the midwife agreed with me.

Emotionally, it was difficult. I cried a lot and was sad for a while afterwards. When I had another period, the feelings of sadness came rushing back, because it brought home the fact that I was no longer pregnant.

At the beginning of this pregnancy, I had been working in a high-stress job (which had only recently become this way because of changes in the company). As a result, I had started drinking soda. When I found out I was pregnant, I stopped and had headaches for the rest of the pregnancy. I quit the stressful job before I miscarried.

I personally believe the caffeine may have been the cause for my miscarriage. However, I'll never know for sure. There are women who drink loads of caffeine and somehow continue through their pregnancies unharmed. But there are also many people who smoke for decades and never get cancer. I have since tried to get over the guilt, because there's nothing I can do to change the past.

Fourth Pregnancy
(Unassisted Birth at Home)

I conceived again about three months after the miscarriage. We weren't actively trying to conceive, but just kind of playing things by ear. Fortunately, we've never had any trouble getting pregnant.

At the beginning of this pregnancy, I had some light bleeding, and I was sure I was going to miscarry again. At ten weeks, I went to the midwife (same midwife as for the third pregnancy), and together, we heard the heartbeat. I had two more prenatal appointments at the same birth center.

The midwife belonged to a group of four, and I had only met two of them by the time I was 20 weeks along. Neither of them acted heartwarmingly friendly. They did some blood work at one appointment and never mentioned it at the next. When I asked for the results, they told me my iron was kind of low, but otherwise, everything was okay. I was annoyed that they obviously would never have told me this if I hadn't asked. What is the point of testing when you don't communicate the results?

The last appointment with the midwife included an ultrasound, where we found out we were having a boy. Shortly before the appointment,

I met a woman who had given birth unassisted to her fourth child. This gave me the push I needed. I had been contemplating unassisted childbirth all along, but I worried my husband wouldn't agree to it.

It took him a while to get used to the idea. But now he knows giving birth is something I end up doing by myself. The midwife may be there for me, but I am the one doing "all the work". He also felt better knowing someone else had given birth unassisted in our area. Somehow this made it seem more realistic for him.

When I had the miscarriage, I was really surprised how my body handled it with no help. It made me think it couldn't be that much harder to have a baby by myself. Besides, the outcome would be a much happier one.

My fourth pregnancy was the longest pregnancy yet. I stopped receiving prenatal care after 20 weeks. At 42 weeks and 2 days, I had a panic attack. I was worried the baby wasn't coming, because he wasn't in the correct position. Specifically, I thought he might be transverse breech. I went to the hospital that day, because I couldn't get a hold of a midwife to do a prenatal appointment. Fortunately, at the hospital, the nurse was helpful. She assured me the baby was fine and his heartbeat sounded great. She also checked my cervix. She could feel the baby's head. She told me I was 2 or 3 cm dilated and 90% effaced.

I had been having contractions on and off for several weeks, so I wasn't surprised my cervix was getting ready. The doctor at the hospital told me he didn't know if the baby was in distress without doing a round of further testing. But it relieved me to know my baby was head down. It was the only thing I had been really concerned about. Therefore, I declined all further testing and went home reassured.

Because of various outside pressures, I felt the need to induce labor. I tried walking, castor oil, sex, and playing with my cervix to induce labor. While almost everything I did caused more Braxton-Hicks contractions, nothing made me go into true labor, even after 42 weeks of pregnancy.

After I passed 43 weeks, even my mother-in-law started talking to me and my husband about going to the hospital. She was concerned with all the usual things associated with a post-term pregnancy (placenta being inadequate, amniotic fluid being too low, etc.).

My husband didn't know what to think. My friend, who had given birth unassisted and is a doula, advised me to find something to do every day that week to get out of the house. On Thursday, we celebrated my oldest daughter's birthday. Afterwards, we left both of our girls at their Grandma's house for a sleepover. That night, I finally gave birth at home. I was 43 weeks and 2 days along.

At midnight, I woke up with contractions and started walking. I really didn't want them to go away as they had before. By 1 a.m., they became quite regular and were 3 minutes apart. At 2.30 a.m., I felt confident I was finally in labor, and I woke up my husband and asked him to get our bedroom ready. He laid out the tarp and blankets and sterilized the umbilical cord scissors. At 2.45 a.m., I had some spotting which excited me greatly, because I felt reassured our baby was ready to join us soon. Around 3 a.m., my husband went into the girls' room to build a Lego house for them. This kept him busy until 4.45 a.m.

During this entire time, I paced the hallway. During each contraction, I would kneel and breathe. I could feel the intensity increasing. My husband's random chatter (he's funny when he's tired) kept me entertained. Around the same time as he was done with Legos, I stopped pacing. I was tired, and I was not afraid the contractions would go away like they had in the past several weeks leading up to this.

Eventually, the pain got more intense, and I couldn't talk during contractions anymore. My husband said they seemed to get closer together, but we never actually timed them. After a while, I started

228

getting the urge to push, and I felt like I really needed to go to the bathroom at the same time. During the entire night, I had gone to the toilet to pee every ten minutes. But it was uncomfortable to be in the bathroom during a contraction.

When the urge to push was irresistible, I started bearing down during the contractions, which now seemed to last forever. I screamed during the pushing stage (same as with my second child), and I think my husband was worried about the neighbors. Pushing didn't last longer than ten minutes, and our baby boy was born at 6.16 a.m. In one contraction before the baby was born, my water broke. It was kind of neat to watch the little waterfall. I also heard and felt the water break. To me, it sounded like a balloon popping.

During the next contraction, I felt his head crowning. Then his head came out, and his entire body followed in one swoop. My husband saw our baby's hand after his head came out. I tried to get a hold of the baby, but he was so slippery I couldn't catch him. He landed on the comforter beneath me, but since I was on my knees with my hands resting on our bed, he didn't fall far at all.

Afterwards, my husband said the personality change in me was amazing. I went from screaming in pain to cooing over the baby within seconds. My husband had a warm towel ready, and we rubbed him and wrapped him in it. Baby Michael cried immediately. Unfortunately, the umbilical cord was short and after a few minutes of cuddling him by my legs without being able to sit up properly, we cut the cord.

Then I got back on all fours to see if the placenta would come out, but it wasn't ready. Instead, I nursed the baby to help the placenta along. It was weird to have the cord hanging out with shoestring attached (that's how my husband had tied it off). I couldn't sit upright comfortably.

Our baby latched on right away, and after he was done nursing, I handed him back to my husband. This time, the placenta came out easily and painlessly. It was interesting to look at, and I checked it out to make sure it was complete. Everything seemed fine, and I decided against keeping it. The original plan had been to put it in the fridge for a day or two, in case we needed to have someone look at it.

I really wanted to cuddle my baby, but I was a mess. I showered to clean up. Afterwards, I went to sit on our bed with plenty of pads under me and cuddled our new baby. During this time, my husband cleaned up, which was really easy to do. He just rolled up the comforters and tarps and put it all in a trash bag. After he came back from the garbage, we realized the umbilical cord scissors accidentally got thrown away with the rest of the stuff. We boiled another pair of scissors to shorten the baby's cord some more. Then we used the clamp we had bought.

This birth experience was really amazing. It was lovely to decide what to do and when. My husband was wonderful. I think it would be difficult to have a baby without someone else there. I didn't have to worry about having things ready or recording the time when our baby was born. He took care of all of it. And it was great to share this miracle with him and to have someone to talk to about it.

Our son Michael only weighed 7 lbs. 10 oz., which seems tiny considering the length of my pregnancy. But the due date I calculated using my menstrual cycle was accurate and confirmed by the ultrasound at 20 weeks. I felt vindicated about waiting and not getting induced at the hospital. Clearly, he was not ready to be born earlier.

In retrospect, I wouldn't try to induce labor again for two reasons: One, it didn't work, anyway. And two, babies will come when they're ready.

Fifth Pregnancy
(Unassisted Pregnancy and Unassisted Birth)

I gave birth to our fourth child at home. This time, we chose not to receive any prenatal care. Therefore, we had no idea about the gender of the baby. It turned out to be a healthy 7 lbs. 11 oz. baby boy. His two big sisters and his big brother are all excited he's finally here. After all, he took long enough, having been born at 43 weeks and 6 days gestation.

Waiting for a Baby

I had been having Braxton Hicks contractions on and off for a few weeks since around the due date. Sometimes, I'd have a terrible pain in my left side, which would travel down into my thigh. However, contractions always petered out, even though they were sometimes fairly regular. My estimated due date based on my menstrual cycle was June 21st. A conception-based due date would have been closer to July 3rd. Either way, baby Timmy didn't really want to make his appearance as early as that. He was born on July 18th.

My previous pregnancy lasted until 43 weeks and 2 days, and this baby wanted to beat my own personal record. During the last week before he was born, I had contractions daily, and they even followed a pattern. However, as soon as I stopped walking, they would fizzle out.

Bloody Show

On Thursday night, my husband and I went to bed. Outside, a storm was building, and it thundered in the distance. I remember complaining to my husband about the baby not coming, and my husband said to tell the universe tonight is the night. I just chuckled, but I really was getting tired of being pregnant for what seemed like an eternity.

Within a few minutes of lying down, I felt a rush of fluids. I went to the bathroom and turned on the light and was surprised to see bloody show. It looked like a lot of blood to me, but in hindsight, it might have been the fact that blood in the water (in the toilet) always looks like a lot more than it is. I didn't have any painful contractions at the time, which added to my confusion. During previous births, I didn't experience bloody show until labor was well under way.

I told my husband, and he got the room ready. This was about 11.30 p.m. Josh wanted me to walk to encourage labor to progress (at least he suggested it), but I was exhausted and just wanted to lie down. I followed my instincts, and I encouraged my husband to go back to sleep.

Finally in Labor

I woke up at about 1 a.m. with more contractions. I felt hungry and had a few bites of toast. Contractions still weren't painful, but I didn't feel sleepy. Between 1 a.m. and 3 a.m., I walked the hallway a bit, boiled scissors, and cuddled my one-year-old, who had woken up from the thunder and lightning. I didn't time the contractions. Eventually, I went back to bed. The bleeding had slowed down, and I wasn't concerned about it. I was confident our baby would come when he was ready.

As soon as I laid down, I had a powerful contraction. After a few more contractions like it, I sat on the toilet, because it felt better. At around 3 a.m., I woke up Josh. He did a good job keeping my mind off the pain by babbling about random things.

Throughout, I had diarrhea. At some point, the pains got more intense, and I knew the end was near. At the same time, I wanted it all to be over. I wanted to stay on the toilet, because this position felt okay, but I didn't really want the baby to be born there.

Timmy Is Born

I moved on all fours onto the floor in our bedroom. After a few rather painful contractions, I felt compelled to go back to the bathroom. I had the urge to push, and I knew it was time for birth. Logically, I should have stayed on the floor, but I felt compelled to go back to the toilet. I felt his head crowning, and my husband helped me off the toilet. He pulled the comforters into the bathroom and helped me down onto the floor. I was pushing and could feel Timmy's head crowning. It was amazing, but really painful at the same time. I whined about the pain, but my husband encouraged me and told me it was almost over. And wasn't it exciting to feel the baby's head?

I felt my perineum stretch around the head. Then the head was born. The next contraction brought out the rest of our baby. Amazingly enough, the placenta followed immediately afterwards. Unfortunately, we didn't take a picture of the placenta, but it looked like a juicy piece of round steak. Timmy started crying within a short amount of time. After a little while, he latched on and nursed.

Eventually, I got up and took a shower while Josh held our baby. We cut the cord a little later, and I cuddled with Timmy while Josh cleaned up the bathroom.

Timmy Meets His Siblings

The kids slept through everything. My daughter Becky was the first one to wake up. We showed her little Timmy, and her eyes got all big and round as she woke up fully. She smiled and said he was cute. Michael woke up next. He was excited and wanted to lie down next to the baby and hug him and kiss him. He was being really careful and gentle, as much as a 21-month-old can be. Melanie was the last one to meet the new baby. Michael already told her about the baby (saying "baby, baby" the entire time) as she walked towards our room, and she was happily staring at him. She also said he was soooo cute.

Sixth Pregnancy
(Third Unassisted Birth)

In December 2016, I unexpectedly got pregnant again. I was simultaneously ecstatic and shocked, but I suspected the pregnancy within a day of conception. With the new baby coming, we had to reschedule the planned visit to my family in Germany to avoid flying during the last trimester.

At the beginning of my pregnancy, I suspected twins, because my belly got big fast. While we were in Germany in the spring, I dreamed I was carrying quadruplets—all boys. The dream along with other uncertainties in my personal life drove me to find reassurance about the baby.

I scheduled an appointment with a German OB/GYN. She performed an ultrasound and confirmed there was only one baby, most likely a girl. I think both the doctor and I were glad I didn't plan to continue prenatal care with her.

Later, I regretted the ultrasound. I had originally tried to find a midwife who could reassure me about the number of babies just using her hands and a stethoscope, but I couldn't find one. I hated that we already knew the sex of the baby ahead of time.

Every pregnancy and birth is different, even if you've given birth several times. This time, I developed varicose veins in my lower right leg. It worried me greatly, because my mother had a thrombosis in her leg. Of course, varicose veins aren't unusual in pregnancy, and my leg didn't hurt.

Braxton Hicks contractions started at 34 weeks of gestation with this baby. Having pre-labor contractions wasn't a novel experience for me, but they had never started this early before. It offered a glimmer of hope maybe this baby would come closer to her due date since this was my first unassisted birth with a girl baby. Supposedly, it's boys who take longer.

At the end of August, about a week before my due date, I woke up with painful contractions. I even woke up my husband and asked him to get the room ready—I was so sure this was it. After a while, the contractions simply stopped.

234

I was disappointed and confused. The next day, I felt let down, because I was still pregnant. I kept having contractions on and off over the next few days. They continued to be rather painful, so much that I had to breathe through them. And yet, my baby didn't want to come.

Braxton-Hicks contractions continued to show up daily, but they were less painful now. This pregnancy also continued past 42 weeks. Apparently, post-term pregnancies are my specialty. But at least, she came before 43 weeks. She was born at 42 weeks and 5 days.

One morning, I woke up with the kids around 7 a.m. Contractions started again, but I didn't pay attention to them. They were my norm. We were working on a shopping list, because my husband had plans to go to the store.

I had to stop in between to breathe deeply through the contractions. My husband asked if he shouldn't stay home. But I was sure the baby wouldn't come anyway, especially if he stayed. But things picked up, and he ended up staying, which was a good thing.

The contractions quickly became more intense. By 8 a.m., I was in the bathroom—my planned birthing location. Our bathroom is spacious, and I liked having the toilet nearby. I actually hopped in the shower, because I hadn't taken one yet. However, my husband had to help me dry off, because I couldn't bend over with the contractions coming on strong. I didn't even bother getting dressed, because I knew birth was imminent.

The birth differed from the others in many ways, especially the time of day. All the kids were awake. We let them watch TV to keep them occupied and out of the way. Meanwhile, my husband sterilized scissors. He thought he had plenty of time, based on his previous experience with my births.

But by this time, I was already in transition, and I yelled for him. He finally came back to me—not fast enough, in my opinion—and stayed. With the other unassisted births, my husband was in the room with me, but I didn't want to be touched. This time, I craved physical contact with him and held onto him. I even had the urge to bite him, because it hurt so much, but I didn't (to his relief).

Then my water broke, and it was green. I was momentarily nervous, but I knew it didn't have to mean anything bad. I worried even as I gave birth to her. But she cried just like the others. I had the feeling she cried harder and longer, but my husband didn't notice any difference compared to our other babies.

As the ultrasound predicted, we had another girl—our tie breaker. She weighed 8 lbs 3 oz. The birth was faster than all the rest. The first contractions happened after 7 a.m. My baby was born at 8.58 a.m. in record time.

I cuddled with her for a while and then took another shower. After I was cleaned up and cuddling with our baby in our bed, we talked about her name. We had several favorites, but in the end, we named her Katelyn, short Katie.

While I gave birth, part of me hoped the other kids would come and watch. I still couldn't decide if I wanted them to be present or not. Later, my oldest told me Michael got scared when he heard me scream. But she told him I was having the baby.

Michael came to look in on us while we were still huddled up in the bathroom. Presumably, he didn't like what he saw, because he didn't stay long. Or maybe the TV was more interesting.

It took a while until the kids came to meet their new sister. I was glad to rest in bed and cuddle with the baby. At the time of this writing, the baby is already 3 ½ years old. By now, she has become an integral part of our family, just like all the rest of them.

Recommended Reading and Resources

A lot of books have been written about childbirth. Most of them focus on traditional medical care during pregnancy and birth, as experienced in our Western World. There are only a few books on homebirths and even fewer on unassisted childbirth. If you're just diving into the topic, you may want to read some other accounts of childbirth. But most of all, trust your instincts and believe in yourself. Your body knows what to do.

Print Resources

"Unassisted Childbirth"
by Laura Kaplan Shanley

The author has given birth to all her children unassisted at home. Her book provides many explanations and examples about the problems and complications caused by medical interventions. Her book also includes an interesting psychological part about the power of your mind and how you can use it to create your own experience. Her book features several birth stories, including her own.

"Ina May's Guide to Childbirth"
by Ina May Gaskin

This is a midwife's account of natural childbirths that happened on "The Farm". Members of this community gave birth at home with a midwife present. Gaskin emphasizes the mind-body-connection and how a healthy lifestyle is necessary to have a healthy birth. Almost half of her book includes inspiring birth stories. She doesn't mention unassisted childbirth, but she emphasizes that childbirth should not be interfered with as is commonly done at the hospital.

"Home Birth On Your Own Terms"
by Heather Baker

This how-to guide on unassisted childbirth covers everything from conception, nutrition, labor, and birth to possible complications and their solutions. Written by a practicing midwife and mother of five, this book includes beautiful pictures and birth stories. If you need directions on the use of herbs and essential oils, including dosage and preparation, this book is a must-have.

"Unassisted Homebirth: An Act of Love"
by Lynn M. Griesemer

This is a book about an unassisted homebirth by someone who has done it. She had four children at the hospital, and the fifth child was born unassisted at home with her husband. Besides birth stories, this book includes many questions and answers by couples who have attempted an unassisted birth. Griesemer doesn't like the interference of midwives and feels strongly about every woman's ability to give birth on her own.

"Emergency Childbirth: A Manual"
by Gregory White

This manual is a mostly positive account of childbirth. There are some worst-case scenarios listed with their consequences, but the author stresses repeatedly how infrequent complications in childbirth are. He mentions that the laboring woman shouldn't eat, which I disagree with (and I'm not the only one), but this doesn't detract from the usefulness of this book.

"The Essential Homebirth Guide: For Families Planning or Considering Birth at Home"
by Jane E. Drichta, Jodilyn Owen, and Dr. Christina Northrup

This book is written for women who are interested in a homebirth. It answers a lot of questions about common illnesses and concerns during pregnancy. The premise of the book is you need to find good midwifery care. Therefore, the authors don't teach you how to give birth on your own, but the book has some excellent information about pregnancy and natural birth.

"The Thinking Woman's Guide to a Better Birth"
by Henci Goer

Henci Goer writes about avoiding interventions in order to have a natural birth. In her book, she stresses the importance of choosing the right provider to increase your chances of giving birth naturally. She also mentions there's never a guarantee for a positive outcome, no matter which option you choose at any given moment. She believes (and I agree) your odds are better without most interventions for pretty much every scenario.

Resources from the Web

I have done extensive research to write this book, much of it online. Whenever I quote or paraphrase a source, I have indicated so on the spot. I list those sources at the end of each chapter. You can find a list of the remaining sources that provided me with a lot of general information here.

The web is an ever-changing resource, and therefore, some links may not work by the time you read this book. Similarly, the content on the sites may have changed from the time I viewed them. You might still find the information by searching for the article titles and authors online. I encourage you to do your own research if you have any questions or concerns about pregnancy, childbirth, or your specific medical needs.

- Agency for Healthcare Research and Quality (2012). "Measuring Your Blood Pressure at Home: A Review of the Research for Adults". Retrieved from http://effectivehealthcare.ahrq.gov/index.cfm/search-for-guides-reviews-and-reports/?productid=894&pageaction=displayproduct.
- American Pregnancy Association (2013). "Group B Strep Infection: GBS." Retrieved from http://americanpregnancy.org/pregnancycomplications/groupbstrepinfection.html.

- American Pregnancy Association (2014). "Water Birth". Retrieved from http://americanpregnancy.org/labornbirth/waterbirth.html.
- BabyCenter, L.L.C. (2012). "Assisted birth (forceps and venthouse)". Retrieved from http://www.babycentre.co.uk/a546719/assisted-birth-forceps-and-ventouse.
- BabyCenter, L.L.C. (2012) "Urine tests during pregnancy". Retrieved from http://www.babycenter.com/0_urine-tests-during-pregnancy_1699.bc?page=1.
- Baby Center L.L.C. (2013) "Frequent urination during pregnancy". Retrieved from http://www.babycenter.com/0_frequent-urination-during-pregnancy_237.bc.
- BabyCenter, L.L.C. (2013). "Giving birth by cesarean section". Retrieved from http://www.babycenter.com/0_giving-birth-by-cesarean-section_160.bc?page=3.
- BabyCenter Medical Advisory Board (2014). "Postpartum hair loss". Retrieved from http://www.babycenter.com/0_postpartum-hair-loss_11721.bc.
- Burgess, Kelly (n.d.) "Pros and Cons of Unassisted Birth". Retrieved from http://www.babyzone.com/pregnancy/labor-and-delivery/unassisted-birth_71600.
- ChangeSurfer Consulting (n.d.). "Episiotomy: Ritual Genital Mutilation in Western Obstetrics" Retrieved from http://www.changesurfer.com/Hlth/episiotomy.html.
- Cherylyn (2010). "Freebirth (Unassisted Childbirth)" Retrieved from http://mamasandbabies.blogspot.de/2010/06/freebirth-unassisted-childbirth.html.
- Doyle, Jennifer, RN, MSN, WHNP-B C (2011). "When is it Time to Push? 'Laboring Down' in Labor and Delivery". Retrieved from http://www.summaflourish.org/2011/07/when-is-it-time-to-push-%E2%80%98laboring-down%E2%80%99-in-labor-and-delivery/.
- Dreynolds (2008). "Antibiotic Eye Ointment in Babies". Retrieved from http://www.smartparentshealthykids.com/blog/?p=912.
- Earhart, Mary (2013). "Alternative treatment to control postpartum bleeding" Retrieved from http://www.ehow.com/way_5814271_alternative-treatment-control-postpartum-bleeding.html.
- Fleiss, Paul M., M.D. (1997). "The Case Against Circumcision" as published in Mothering: Magazine of Natural Family Living. Retrieved from http://www.mothersagainstcirc.org/fleiss.html.

- GivingBirthNaturally.com (2012). "Understanding The Stages of Labor". Retrieved from http://www.givingbirthnaturally.com/stages-of-labor.html.
- Goldberg, Carey (2013). "Tragically Wrong: When Good Early Pregnancies Are Misdiagnosed As Bad." Retrieved from http://commonhealth.wbur.org/2013/10/ectopic-pregnancy-misdiagnosed-methotrexate
- Gray, Kimberly (2012). "Some area women choosing natural childbirth" Retrieved from http://www.reporternews.com/news/2012/jun/25/some-area-women-choosing-natural-childbirth/.
- Grayson, Charlotte (2005). "Giving Birth the Old Way" Retrieved from http://www.medicinenet.com/script/main/art.asp?articlekey=51649.
- Harkins, Don (1999). "National standard mandates newborn vitamin K injection" Retrieved from http://www.proliberty.com/observer/19990710.htm.
- Haskell, Christie (2011). "What's With the Eye Ointment Put in Newborn's Eyes?" Retrieved from http://thestir.cafemom.com/pregnancy/117351/Whats_With_the_Eye_Ointment.
- Intact America (2013). "The Facts behind Circumcision" Retrieved from http://www.intactamerica.org/learnmore.
- Kiely & Kogan, (n. d.) "Reproductive Health of Women – Prenatal Care". Retrieved from http://www.cdc.gov/reproductivehealth/ProductsPubs/DatatoAction/pdf/rhow8.pdf
- Kohle, Diana. "Umbilical Cord Prolapse" Copyright by EBSCO Publishing. Retrieved from http://www.lifescript.com/health/a-z/conditions_a-z/conditions/u/umbilical_cord_prolapse.aspx.
- Kresser (2011). "Natural childbirth IIb: ultrasound not as safe as commonly thought". Retrieved from http://chriskresser.com/natural-childbirth-iib-ultrasound-not-as-safe-as-commonly-thought.
- Laskowski, M.D. (2013) "What's a normal resting heart rate?" Retrieved from http://www.mayoclinic.com/health/heart-rate/AN01906.
- Makulec, Amanda (2012). "Every Birthday Starts with the Golden Minute". Retrieved from http://blog.usaid.gov/2012/04/every-birthday-starts-with-the-golden-minute/.
- Mama Birth (2012). "A Little Postpartum Surprise: Afterpains!" Retrieved from http://mamabirth.blogspot.com/2012/04/little-postpartum-surprise-afterpains.html.

- Martin JA, Hamilton BE, Ventura SJ, et al. Births: Final data for 2010. National vital statistics reports; vol 61 no 1. Hyattsville, M.D.: National Center for Health Statistics. 2012.

- Martin, Piper (2013). "Homeopathic Remedies to treat Hemorrhage". Retrieved from http://midwifeinternational.org/how-to-become-midwife/homeopathic-remedies-treat-hemorrhage/.

- Mayo Clinic (2013). "Labor and delivery, postpartum care" Retrieved from http://www.mayoclinic.com/health/stages-of-labor/PR00106.

- Mayo Foundation for Medical Education and Research (2014). "Signs of labor: Know what to expect." Retrieved from http://www.mayoclinic.org/healthy-living/labor-and-delivery/in-depth/signs-of-labor/art-20046184?pg=1.

- Mercola, Dr. (2010). "The Dark Side of the Routine Newborn Vitamin K Shot". Retrieved from http://articles.mercola.com/sites/articles/archive/2010/03/27/high-risks-to-your-baby-from-vitamin-k-shot-they-dont-warn-you-about.aspx.

- Myers, Lucy (2007). "Is Unassisted Childbirth Legal?" Retrieved from http://voices.yahoo.com/is-unassisted-childbirth-legal-537163.html?cat=52.

- Natural Motherhood (2012). "Internal and External Fetal Monitoring Risks." Retrieved from http://www.natural-motherhood.com/external-fetal-monitoring.html.

- New Zealand College of Midwives (2010) "The vaginal examination during labour: is it of benefit or harm?" Retrieved from http://www.thefreelibrary.com/The+vaginal+examination+during+labour%3A+is+it+of+benefit+or+harm%3F-a0251277462

- Reed, Rachel (2010). "Nuchal Cords: the perfect scapegoat" Retrieved from http://midwifethinking.com/2010/07/29/nuchal-cords/.

- Robertson, Andrea (1998). "If your baby is breech" Retrieved from https://www.birthinternational.com/articles/midwifery/37-if-your-baby-is-breech.

- Romano, A. (2009). "First, Do No Harm: How Routine Interventions, Common Restrictions, and the Organization of Our Health-Care System Affect the Health of Mothers and Newborns". From the journal of perinatal education. Retrieved from http://www.ncbi.nlm.nih.gov/pmc/articles/PMC2730908/.

- Sanger, Jeff (2012). "Should I circumcise? Top Ten Reasons Circumcision Sucks." Retrieved from http://shouldicircumcise.blogspot.de/2012/06/top-ten-reasons-circumcision-sucks.html.

- Schalken, Lara (2013). "Birth Customs Around the World." Retrieved from http://www.parents.com/pregnancy/giving-birth/vaginal/birth-customs-around-the-world/?page=1.

- Terreri, Cara (2011). "Postpartum Care: "After Pains"." Retrieved from http://givingbirthwithconfidence.org/2011/11/postpartum-care-after-pains/.

- Terreri, Cara (2014). "Why You May Want to "Labor Down" Before Pushing in Birth." Retrieved from http://givingbirthwithconfidence.org/2014/01/why-you-may-want-to-labor-down-before-pushing-in-birth/.

- The Center for Unhindered Living (2006). "Do-It-Yourself Prenatal Care" Retrieved from http://www.unhinderedliving.com/prenatal.html.

- The Center for Unhindered Living (2009). "Newborn Procedures". Retrieved from http://www.unhinderedliving.com/newborn.html.

- The Center for Unhindered Living (2001). "Newborn Eye Ointment – Is it necessary and effective?" Retrieved from http://www.unhinderedliving.com/eyeointment.html.

- The Deranged Housewife (2010). "Do-It-Yourself Pregnancy" Retrieved from http://thederangedhousewifeonline.blogspot.de/2010/04/do-it-yourself-pregnancy.html.

- Todd, Nivin, M.D., FACOG (2012). "Can Labor Be Induced Naturally?" Retrieved from http://www.webmd.com/baby/inducing-labor-naturally-can-it-be-done?page=2

- Vogel, Lauren (2011). "'Do it yourself' births prompt alarm" Retrieved from http://www.ncbi.nlm.nih.gov/pmc/articles/PMC3071383/.

- Weiss, Robin Elise (2011). "Episiotomy – Is it really necessary?" Retrieved from http://pregnancy.about.com/cs/episiotomy/a/aa042897.htm.

- Weiss, Robin Elise, LCCE (2013). "How is Pitocin used to induce labor?" Retrieved from http://pregnancy.about.com/od/induction/f/pitocin.htm.

- Weiss, Robin Elise, LCCE (2013). "Unassisted Birth" Retrieved from http://pregnancy.about.com/cs/unassistedbirth/a/aa080999.htm.

- Weiss, Robin Elise, LCCE (2013). "Pitocin FAQ" Retrieved from http://www.childbirth.org/articles/pit.html.

Printed in Great Britain
by Amazon